How to Get that

Training Post in Ophthalmology

The E

Ophth

Secon

Brian A

Consulta

Royal Vi

Melbour

Shi Zhu

Academ

North W

Manche

Ken Le

Ophthal

West of

Glasgow

HOW TO GET THAT TRAINING POST IN OPHTHALMOLOGY
Second Edition

Table of Contents

Forewords

Despite political, climatic and financial upheaval all around us, medicine still remains one of the best careers and ophthalmology, combining both medicine and surgery, is the jewel in the crown.

Many still consider it as a Cinderella specialty, but this may be because they have never worked out which way up to hold an ophthalmoscope and are put off by the incomprehensible array of acronyms in ophthalmology notes.

I feel embarrassed to admit that after doing a combined surgical and ophthalmology house job I was given a recommendation to visit a unit on the South coast and meet the boss. I went. He shook my hand, told me to read all twelve volumes of Duke Elder, twice, and walked me over to Medical staffing and said "Sign here; you've got the job!"

Things have changed a little since those days! Many others have seen the light and realise the potential of going into ophthalmology. The competition is keen. However, don't give up – read this marvellous guide and you will be equipped with more knowledge of how to achieve your goal than has ever been collated before. Just don't show it to anyone else!

Mr. Nick Astbury FRCS, FRCOphth, FRCP
President of the Royal College of Ophthalmologists, 2003-2006
Chair VISION 2020 United Kingdom
Consultant Ophthalmic Surgeon
Department of Ophthalmology
Norfolk & Norwich University Hospital NHS Trust
Norwich, United Kingdom

Ophthalmology is a competitive specialty with a high level of satisfaction among colleagues. Perhaps it is not surprising we are able to attract such bright students year after year. Sight is a precious gift. Being able to restore or prevent blindness is an enormous responsibility and a privilege, because the impact in quality of life is very large. Ours is a rapidly evolving specialty and we are now fortunate to enjoy very effective treatments, sophisticated diagnostic technologies, and we certainly are the very best of surgeons, operating under a microscope and manipulating delicate tissues of a few microns of thickness.

If you want to be an ophthalmologist, do follow carefully the useful advice that Dr. Ang and colleagues are offering you. I am certain that it will be very helpful, and we hope to welcome you to our world in the very near future.

Professor Augusto Azuara-Blanco PhD, FRCS(Ed), FRCOphth
Clinical Professor
Centre for Vision and Vascular Science
School of Medicine, Dentistry and Biomedical Sciences
Belfast, United Kingdom

This handbook intends to unravel the intricacies of ophthalmic training in the United Kingdom. It is obvious that in a competitive specialty like ophthalmology, planning should begin preferably at the undergraduate level. This book sheds some light on the career pathway that recent and current United Kingdom ophthalmology trainees would have undergone for entry into ophthalmic specialty training. In addition, it highlights the problems faced by many trainees and provides possible solutions to them.

The authors must be congratulated for putting together this handbook, which is a welcome addition to any ophthalmology bibliography. It provides well-articulated information that is essential for those who plan to pursue a career in ophthalmology.

Lastly, although this book is targeted for those in the United Kingdom, it will also be useful for those in similar situations in the rest of the British Commonwealth since postgraduate training in many of these countries is loosely based on the United Kingdom training curriculum in ophthalmology.

Professor Visvaraja Subrayan MBBS, FRCS(E), FRCOphth(UK), AM
Department of Ophthalmology
Faculty of Medicine
University of Malaya
Kuala Lumpur, Malaysia

Reviews of First Edition

I've often been asked for advice about how to go about putting in an effective application – and often finished wondering if I've included everything that might help. Well, now I can direct people to How to Get that Training Post in Ophthalmology.

Ms Lucilla Butler

Consultant Ophthalmologist

Former Chair of the West Midlands Training Committee, United Kingdom

This book may not guarantee you an ophthalmology job, but it sure will help!

Professor Baljean Dhillon

NES Personal Chair of Clinical Ophthalmology

University of Edinburgh, United Kingdom

The guide contains a wealth of invaluable advice, complemented by a consistently extensive resource list in each chapter. There is a great deal of generic information and guidance contained therein which will prove invaluable to junior doctors competing for training posts in any specialty.

Mr Mark Daniel Doherty

Ophthalmic Trainees' Group

Royal College of Ophthalmologists, United Kingdom

Read this book if you are interested in joining the field of ophthalmology in the UK. In fact, if you are just interested in becoming an elite candidate in any field in any country, you can extrapolate the advice for any career.

Dr Damien Luviano

Chief of Ophthalmology

Joslin Diabetes Center, United States of America

This lively and informative book is a must-read for all aspiring ophthalmologists. I only wish I had access to such a book when I was a medical student.

Dr Habiba Saedon

Ophthalmology Specialty Trainee

West Midlands Deanery, United Kingdom

Preface

Ophthalmology is no longer the 'hidden' specialty it once was. In the not-too-distant past, only a handful of medical students would think of, much less consider, a career in ophthalmology. The recent advances in medical therapeutics, imaging technology, and surgical techniques and equipment have brought ophthalmology to the forefront of the public eye. These exciting developments, coupled with the increasing importance of work-life balance, now make ophthalmology one of the most sought after specialties in the United Kingdom and the rest of the world. Competition for ophthalmology posts, both training and non-training, has never been higher. This in itself can be very daunting to someone who wants to enter into ophthalmology, but **does not know HOW to do so**. This is very apparent in the questions that we have been asked over and over again: "How do I get into ophthalmology? What do I need to do to get an ophthalmology post?"

It is the intention of this book to **show** and **guide** prospective ophthalmic trainees, step-by-step, how to achieve their aim of getting into ophthalmology. While this guide is primarily aimed for those wishing to train in the United Kingdom, the principles should hold true for any training programme anywhere in the world. True, it will require plenty of hard work and perseverance – and with the correct guidance, you **WILL succeed**!

Good luck!

Brian Ang
Shi Zhuan Tan
Ken Lee Lai
http://ophthalmologytraining.blogspot.com

Acknowledgements

The second edition of this book is the culmination of more hard work and long nights in researching, reading, interviewing, discussing, writing, editing and project managing. We would certainly not have been able to do it without the unstinting assistance, encouragement, advice and guidance provided by our family, friends and colleagues while writing this book.

In particular, we would like to thank Lindsey Lee, Madam K.L. Ooi, Winnie W.N., Bhuma Paranjothy, Janet Paget and Professor Chung Nen Chua for their contributions and support in coming up with this second edition.

Finally, we hope that you will enjoy reading and learning from this book as much as we have writing it!

Chapter 1

Ophthalmology as a Specialty

Brian Ang

Shi Zhuan Tan

Ophthalmology as a Specialty

Pros:

- Exciting mix of medicine and surgery
- Very interesting – has its fair share of diagnostic dilemmas
- Challenging microsurgery
- High job satisfaction by helping patients gain a better quality of life
- No deaths (unless from very rare and unforeseen circumstances)
- Great on-calls (comparatively speaking), with few or no in-patients
- Being able to work anywhere – your main job can be combined with overseas work, such as with the Vision 2020 links programme: https://www.iceh.org.uk/display/WEB/VISION+2020+Links+programme

Cons:

- Busy (sometimes ridiculously so) out-patient clinics
- Consultation time can be lengthy for some patients, particularly when dealing with social issues related to poor sight
- Registering patients as blind / partially sighted

Problems:

- VERY competitive
- Not everyone is good at it
- Stereopsis and good hand-eye co-ordination imperative
- Poor exposure in medical school
- Political – lack of jobs, lack of surgical time, increasing subspecialism

In the UK, the pursuit of streamlining training posts and ensuring run-through training via *Modernising Medical Careers* (*MMC* – http://www.mmc.nhs.uk) has resulted in major consequences:

- Firstly, this resulted in a significant reduction in the number of training posts. Effectively, all the previous *Senior House Officer (SHO)* posts have been wiped out, with only 50% of the previously available training posts remaining. As a result, service provision and duties and tasks traditionally done by the SHO are now being performed by the *Specialist Registrars (SpR) / Specialty Registrars (StRs)*, whose duties in turn are increasingly taken over by the consultant.

- Secondly, the run-through training has been achieved at the expense of flexibility. Trainees no longer have the flexibility to switch between SHO posts – this used to be advantageous in the past as trainees would be able to sample the various specialties for 6-month periods before deciding on a career choice. SHOs used to have the option of gaining experience in allied specialties, such as neurology or rheumatology, but this is now becoming more difficult.

- Finally, MMC has pushed competitive entry to a much earlier stage. In the past, the bottleneck used to be at the SHO level, where many SHOs, after passing their entry exams, would compete against each other for the coveted SpR post. Trainees would use their 2 to 4 years in the SHO grade to gain valuable clinical and surgical skills, conduct audits, undertake research projects, attend courses and present at conferences, all to beef up their CV to the standard required for shortlisting for SpR posts. The CV boosting period was, on average, of around 4 years' duration after graduating from medical school. Now, with MMC, applications for OST posts are due only a few months after the start of *Foundation Year 2 (FY2)*. In other words, newly qualified doctors only have approximately *18 months after graduation* to improve their CVs to the previous SpR-equivalent standard.

A training post in ophthalmology equips the trainee with specialist clinical and surgical skills specific to ophthalmology. Once in an **Ophthalmology Specialty Training (OST)** programme, the trainee obtains a National Training Number (NTN) and must fulfil all the training requirements of the **Royal College of Ophthalmologists** (http://curriculum.rcophth.ac.uk) to progress, and also pass postgraduate examinations. At the end of OST, you will receive a **Certificate of Completion of Training (CCT)**, which enables you to apply for consultant posts in the United Kingdom (UK).

- **Clinical ophthalmology**

  Ophthalmology Specialty Training (OST) is a "run-through" training programme, where progression to the next level is automatic as long as all competency requirements are satisfied. Most programmes span 7 years, with rotations through the major ophthalmic subspecialties. Most trainees spend an extra year or more doing fellowships in the subspecialty of their choice, either locally or abroad. This can be done after the CCT has been obtained or during training, in which case approval is required from the Postgraduate Deanery and the Royal College of Ophthalmologists. The process to become a consultant will take 8 to 9 years, possibly 10 or more.

- **Academic ophthalmology**

  You may pursue an academic training post in ophthalmology, via the **Academic Clinical Fellowship (ACF)**. The ACFs in ophthalmology developed by the **National Institute for Health Research (NIHR)** usually take 3 years, followed by the **Research Training Fellowship (RTF)** for 3 to 4 years, leading to a PhD (or equivalent). Thereafter, a **Clinical Lectureship (CL)** beckons, typically with 50% research time and 50% clinical time, until the attainment of the CCT several years later. The CCT allows for the application for senior lecturer posts, and after a good number of years (and a multitude of research publications later), the title of "Professor" may finally be achieved!

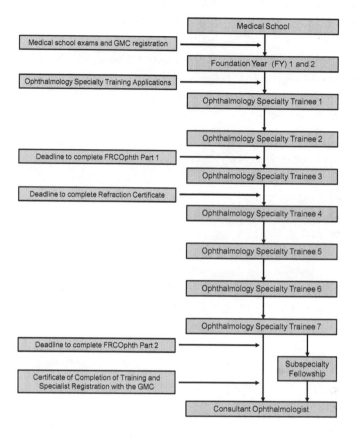

Figure 1: Pathway for Ophthalmology Specialty Training (OST) in the UK

Ophthalmology Specialty Training Assessments

Progression of OST from one year to the next is contingent upon achieving the specific learning outcomes for the year. The learning outcomes are based on the OST curriculum set by the Royal College of Ophthalmologists (http://curriculum.rcophth.ac.uk), and consist of 180 learning outcomes in 13 domains of clinical practice. Progression is assessed through the Portfolio, Annual Review of Competence Progression (ARCP) and Workplace Based Assessments (WpBA).

- **Portfolio**

  http://curriculum.rcophth.ac.uk/assessments/portfolio

  The training portfolio is an important way for the trainee to collect evidence that learning outcomes have been met in the course of OST. The portfolio is used to record the following:
  - Work-place based assessments
  - Logbook of procedures and clinical cases
  - Reflective diary, including current clinical experience and learning plan
  - Appraisal documents, such as meetings with the educational supervisor
  - Revalidation and annual assessment
  - Continuous professional development, both formal and informal
  - Audit, research and teaching activities
  - Clinical governance issues, such as critical incidents, complaints, guidelines

- **Annual Review of Competence Progression (ARCP)**

  http://curriculum.rcophth.ac.uk/assessments/rita_guide

  The ARCP is a yearly review of the specific learning outcomes that the trainee has achieved during the past OST year. This provides the opportunity to scrutinise and document the trainee's progression, and to flag any areas for improvement. The trainee can only progress to the next year of OST subject to satisfactory completion of competencies as determined at the ARCP.

- **Workplace-Based Assessments (WpBA)**

  http://curriculum.rcophth.ac.uk/assessments/wba

  Various WpBA tools have been developed to assess the trainee and to provide evidence of acceptable performance in the various learning outcome domains. These tools and their learning outcome domains are listed below:

  - *Clinical Rating Scale (CRS)*

    Learning outcome domains: clinical assessment; practical refraction

  - *Case-based Discussion (CbD)*

    Learning outcome domains: patient investigation; information handling; communication; attitudes; ethics and responsibilities; decision making; clinical reasoning and judgement; role in the health service; continuing personal and professional development

  - *Direct Observation of Procedural Skills (DOPS)*

    Learning outcome domains: practical skills; communication

  - *Objective Assessment of Surgical and Technical Skills (OSATS)*

    Learning outcome domains: practical skills; communication

  - *Multi-Source Feedback (MSF)*

    Learning outcome domains: communication; information handling; attitudes; ethics and responsibilities; clinical reasoning and judgement; role in health service; decision making; continuing personal and professional development

Ophthalmology Examination Structure

In the course of Ophthalmic Specialty Training, you will be expected to sit and pass written and clinical examinations set by the Royal College of Ophthalmologists. These are the FRCOphth Part 1, Refraction Certificate, and FRCOphth Part 2. Trainees must pass FRCOphth Part 1 by the end of OST2, the Refraction Certificate by the end of OST3, and FRCOphth Part 2 by OST7. All trainees have a maximum of *6 attempts to pass each examination*.

- **FRCOphth Part 1 (Written)**
    - Multiple choice questions (120 questions; 3 hours)
    - Constructed response question (12 questions; 2 hours)
    - Topics examined:
        - ✓ Anatomy – orbit and adnexae, ocular anatomy, cranial cavity, central nervous system, head and neck, cardiovascular system
        - ✓ Physiology – general and ocular physiology, physiology of vision
        - ✓ Biochemistry and cell biology
        - ✓ Pathology – general principles, basic ocular pathology, microbiology, immunology
        - ✓ Growth and senescence
        - ✓ Optics – physical and geometric optics, clinical optics
        - ✓ Therapeutics and Pharmacology
        - ✓ Lasers
        - ✓ Epidemiology and Evidence based medicine
        - ✓ Instrument technology
        - ✓ Biostatistics
        - ✓ Clinical genetics
        - ✓ Patient investigations

- **Refraction Certificate (Practical)**
    - Objective structured clinical examination (4 stations; 1 hour)
    - Topics examined:
        - ✓ Retinoscopy
        - ✓ Subjective refraction
        - ✓ Focimetry
        - ✓ Spectacle prescription

- **FRCOphth Part 2 (Written and practical)**
    - Multiple choice questions (90 questions; 2 hours)
    - Extended matching questions (45 2-stem questions; 3 hours)
    - Structured viva (5 stations; 50 minutes)
      Topics examined in the structured viva:
        - ✓ Station 1: Patient investigations and data interpretation (10 minutes)
        - ✓ Station 2; Patient management (10 minutes)
        - ✓ Station 3: Health promotion and disease prevention (10 minutes)
        - ✓ Station 4: Attitudes, ethics and responsibilities (10 minutes)
        - ✓ Station 5: Audit, research and evidence based practice (10 minutes)
    - Clinical examination (6 stations; 1 hour 40 minutes)
      Topics examined in the clinical examination:
        - ✓ Cataract and anterior segment (15 minutes)
        - ✓ Glaucoma and lid (15 minutes)
        - ✓ Posterior segment (15 minutes)
        - ✓ Strabismus and orbit (15 minutes)
        - ✓ Medicine and neurology (30 minutes)
        - ✓ Communication skills (10 minutes)

Additional Careers Information

To learn more about ophthalmology as a career and to gain a better appreciation of the working life of an ophthalmologist, please visit the following websites:

- http://www.rcophth.ac.uk/page.asp?section=321&sectionTitle=Undergraduate+Ophthalmology

- http://careers.bmj.com/careers/advice/view-article.html?id=921

- http://careers.bmj.com/careers/advice/view-article.html?id=1870#

- http://student.bmj.com/student/view-article.html?id=sbmj0207234

- http://www.medicalcareers.nhs.uk/specialty_pages/ophthalmology.aspx

- http://www.ranzco.edu/index.php/component/content/article/49-unused/about-ranzco/51-what-is-an-opthalmologist?Itemid=178

- http://www.aao.org/careers/envision

Chapter 2

Improving Your CV

Brian Ang
Shi Zhuan Tan
Ken Lee Lai

Improving Your CV

Let's face it: the great majority of us are not going to win any Olympic medals or hold any world records. We have all gone through the same process: sixth form (A-levels), medical school, house officer or foundation year jobs. Some may have had previous related or unrelated work experience, but we all still generally appear homogenous from the curriculum vitae (CV) point of view.

The key therefore, is to make ourselves stand out from the crowd. However, how do we achieve this? How can we make ourselves known to the people that matter? What can we do to help us nail that ophthalmology training post?

There are several ways that this can be done, and these will be described in greater detail in the subsections below:

- Choose your mentors
- Study (really) hard during your medical school undergraduate years
- Select your House Officer / Foundation Year posts carefully, and then work (really really) hard
- Participate in audit and research
- Attend, or better yet, present at conferences
- Attend ophthalmology-related courses and workshops
- Attend miscellaneous (non-ophthalmology) courses
- Sit for relevant examinations
- Get involved in ophthalmic charity work
- Contribute to the local ophthalmology department / university

If you want to be an ophthalmologist, you must be prepared to work harder than your peers, and even to work on your vacation days and off-days. There are no shortcuts – this is the only way to build a competitive CV.

Choosing Your Mentors

Choosing mentors is generally not something that people think about because it is not something that can be placed in the CV (apart from the reference section). Given that references are no longer considered the way they used to in the UK, especially when applying for OST posts, it is therefore unsurprising that this is not given due priority. However, it is still arguably one of the most important steps that you can make when deciding to embark upon a career in ophthalmology.

Why? Well, having mentors confers these advantages:

- Source of moral support
- Source of clinical and non-clinical advice and practical tips
- Introductions to other ophthalmologists
- Assistance / ideas with audit and research
- Non-NHS opportunities (local or otherwise)
- Reference – still important in the international context

There is no limit to the number of mentors that you can have. Ideally, at least one of your mentors should be a consultant ophthalmologist; better still if this mentor has a high profile nationally and internationally. It is of utmost importance for you to have some kind of affinity with your mentors, and that they are able to help and guide you to achieve your aims. There is no point in having a mentor whom you have personality clashes with, even if he / she is one of the foremost ophthalmology experts in the world.

Arrange to meet several consultant ophthalmologists, and then approach the ones you feel would be best suited to become your mentors. Most will be happy to take on the role if their circumstances allow, especially if they feel they get along well with you. Remember that this is a two-way relationship – you should strive to avoid anything that may endanger the rapport that you have with your mentors.

Medical School Undergraduate Years

Prior to MMC, displaying an interest in ophthalmology at the undergraduate level was desirable for career progression. Now, this has become virtually essential. As such, prospective trainees are advised to work on their CV while still in medical school. Although likely to impinge upon your medical student social lifestyle, building up your CV early during your student days will give you a definite edge when you eventually apply for OST posts.

- **Distinctions / Prizes / Medals / Bursaries**

  Try to get distinctions, obtain bursaries and win academic prizes / medals throughout your undergraduate years as these will make your CV look very impressive. Most medical schools have an ophthalmology prize / medal up for grabs annually. Enquire at the administrative office of your medical school for lists of internal and external prizes / bursaries that you can apply and compete for.

- **Electives**

  This is an obvious way to improve your CV. Your medical elective can be done either locally or abroad. Aim to spend some time in renowned eye units, such as *Moorfields Eye Hospital* in London or *Wills Eye Hospital* in Philadelphia. These will require forward planning in advance. Decide if you prefer a clinical or research based elective. Do not be afraid to approach professors / consultant ophthalmologists in these departments by email in the first instance to state your intention. If they do not get back to you, show perseverance by contacting the secretary and leaving a message. Contact details (email and telephone numbers) can be easily obtained these days from any internet search engine or from the correspondence details found in their published work in ophthalmology journals. A good reference by your local consultant ophthalmologist will also make applications for competitive elective posts easier. Start making enquiries *at least 1 year in advance*, particularly if going to countries where visas need to be issued.

- **Elective Bursaries / Grants**

  Most medical schools have local bursaries to help medical students with the cost of electives, usually in exchange for a report on how the funds were used. You can also apply for external grants from various medical and charity organisations. Applications are competitive, and you will have to demonstrate why you deserve the bursary / grant. In general, aim to show that the main purpose for your elective is to learn (e.g. from renowned centres) or to contribute (e.g. eye camp in a developing country) rather than to have a holiday abroad – this makes your application more favourable. Travel grants look great on the CV because they demonstrate interest and good planning skills.

  External grants include:
  - *Royal College of Ophthalmologists Patrick Trevor-Roper Award*
    http://www.rcophth.ac.uk/page.asp?section=320&sectionTitle=Awards+and+Prizes

  - *Royal College of Surgeons of Edinburgh Elective Bursaries*
    http://www.rcsed.ac.uk/fellows-members/awards-and-grants/bursaries.aspx

  - *Royal Society of Medicine Student Awards*
    http://www.rsm.ac.uk/academ/awards/index.php

  - *Wellcome Trust Student Elective prize*
    http://www.wellcome.ac.uk/Funding/Biomedical-science/Funding-schemes/PhD-funding-and-undergraduate-opportunities/index.htm

- **Special Study Modules (SSM)**

  Different medical schools have different SSM structures. In general, SSMs involve a period of time learning / researching subjects of your own choosing. Concentrating your SSMs on ophthalmology-related topics demonstrates your keen interest in ophthalmology and enhances your ophthalmic knowledge.

- **Duke Elder Undergraduate Ophthalmology Prize**

  http://www.rcophth.ac.uk/page.asp?section=321&sectionTitle=Undergraduate+Ophthalmology

  This is an annual competitive national extended matching question examination run by the Royal College of Ophthalmologists. Previously seen as desirable, it is now almost a must. Aim to achieve a good position (top 20). It should be sufficient to revise from the basic medical student ophthalmology books, such as *ABC of Eyes* or *Lecture Notes in Ophthalmology*. Other useful learning resources include OphthoBook (http://www.ophthobook.com) and the *International Council of Ophthalmology Handbook for Medical Students* (http://www.icoph.org/pdf/ICOMedicalStudentEnglish.pdf). While there is only one sitting per year, there is no limit to how many years you can take the examination while still a medical student.

- **BSc in an ophthalmology-related field**

  Related fields include *neuroscience*, *visual science* and *ocular imaging technology*. While this option will not suit everyone due to the extra costs involved, it nevertheless provides several advantages. It gives exposure to research (usually laboratory-based) along with all its attendant challenges and frustrations. It also provides the opportunity to apply for funding and research grants. If conducted well, it may also lead to presentations at conferences or even publications in peer-reviewed journals. Doing a BSc potentially provides 4 valuable extra lines in your CV at the cost of only one extra year (BSc, research grant, presentation and publication).

- **Evaluate stereopsis**

  This is important because an ophthalmologist needs to have fine depth perception for routine clinical work as well as microsurgery. Stereopsis can be assessed in a variety of methods, and these are usually performed by orthoptists. Contact your local eye department to (politely) request an evaluation of your stereopsis by an orthoptist.

- **British Undergraduate Ophthalmology Society**

  http://www.buos.co.uk

  The British Undergraduate Ophthalmology Society (BUOS) is a UK-wide ophthalmology society specifically set up as a learning resource for medical students and junior doctors. With BUOS, you will have access to ophthalmology e-learning materials (podcasts, revision notes, lectures), courses (practical ophthalmology skills, Specialty Training interview skills, Specialty Training application skills), education projects and fundraisers. The Annual Student and Trainee Ophthalmology Conference organised by BUOS is a great opportunity to network with like-minded individuals and to learn more about a career in ophthalmology via lectures and workshops.

- **British Undergraduate Journal of Ophthalmology**

  http://www.buos.co.uk/bujo

  The British Undergraduate Journal of Ophthalmology (BUJO) is the official journal of the BUOS. It is an online, peer-reviewed, open access journal that features not only ophthalmology case reports and research, but also articles on careers, education and electives. The elective reports are a great source of ideas and practical information, and are particularly helpful if you are in the process of deciding and planning what to do and where to go for your medical student elective.

House Officer / Foundation Years

Most UK graduates will enter a 2-year Foundation Training programme with no difficulties, although some Postgraduate Deaneries are more competitive than others. The first few months of working as a Foundation Year (FY) doctor will undoubtedly be stressful, as no one is truly prepared for the transition from being a medical student to a junior doctor. That stress, coupled with the potentially unsociable hours, means that future OST applicants often do not have the motivation or time to do anything else apart from work. Nevertheless, it is still important to keep working hard and to keep the momentum going.

Academic Foundation Training is a recent initiative designed to introduce talented newly-qualified foundation doctors to academic research and to provide opportunities for them to acquire the skills necessary to contribute to medical research programmes. It is an excellent stepping stone toward the pursuit of an academic career, and it looks very good on the CV.

- **Choice of posts**

  The best would be to choose an FY programme that includes 4 months in ophthalmology. This provides exposure to working life as an ophthalmologist, and to the clinical evaluation and management of ophthalmic patients (http://careers.bmj.com/careers/advice/view-article.html?id=1870#). Not all Postgraduate Deaneries offer this option, so do consider rotations that include *Accident & Emergency, Neurology, Rheumatology, Endocrinology,* or *Neurosurgery*

  If you do manage to enter an FY2 programme with ophthalmology, you will in all likelihood be doing most of the ward work, and so you may feel somewhat dispirited that you are not seeing as many eyes as you would like. Always try to show enthusiasm and interest – see patients on your own and read up on cases that you've seen that day. You can learn a lot even if you only read about one case each day. Your seniors are definitely also more likely to want to teach someone who is keen and enthusiastic.

- **Taster week**

  Most FY programmes allow up to 10 days of taster in a specialty of your choice so that you have an idea of what that specialty is about. This is usually organised through the local Postgraduate Deanery and is part of the study leave allowance. Doing your taster week in ophthalmology earns you that extra point in your CV and also gives you a chance to establish a relationship with local ophthalmologists.

- **Clinic and theatre experience**

  It will be beneficial to spend some time attending ophthalmology clinics and theatre sessions as an observer. This may necessitate coming in during leave days. This can be arranged either through your mentors or the ophthalmology department secretary. Reading up beforehand ensures that you're not entirely clueless when questioned. It is also a great way to create a good impression.

- **Clinical skills**

  Your résumé appears stronger if you are able to demonstrate that you have basic ophthalmology examination skills, including:

  - *Extraocular muscle movement evaluation*
  - *Assessment of visual fields by confrontation*
  - *Slit lamp biomicroscopy*
  - *Goldmann applanation tonometry*
  - *Direct ophthalmoscopy*

  For an introduction to these topics, visit the *Success in MRCOphth* website (http://www.mrcophth.com) or read Jack Kanski's *Clinical Ophthalmology*. However, clinical skills are learnt not just by reading, but also by observing and being observed. A very good way to learn is by shadowing the on-call ophthalmologist outside working hours. When seeing patients out of hours, there is less pressure on time, and hence more time to be taught these skills. This can usually be arranged through the ophthalmology department secretary or directly with the on-call ophthalmology doctor.

Audit / Research

There is great difficulty in this respect for those wishing to start out in ophthalmology. Randomised controlled trials and case-control studies are impressive in the CV, but take several years to complete and are realistically out of reach for most FY doctors who do not normally remain at one hospital for more than 1 year. Ethics approval is another issue as it can take up to 6 months from application to actual approval. Most peer-reviewed journals now require ethics approval before a manuscript is considered for publication.

- **Case reports**

    Case reports are easier to write up and do not need ethics approval, although patient consent must be obtained. However, cases with interesting learning points (i.e. publishable cases) are not easy to come by. Your mentors and other consultant ophthalmologists may have a case or two that they have not yet had the chance to report – offer to write up the case and prepare it for journal submission. Most journals will have a 'Letter to Editor' or 'Correspondence' section for case reports, but the higher impact journals generally do not accept case reports unless they are of exceptional value.

    Journals that tend to favour case reports include:
    - *BMC Ophthalmology* (requires payment)
      http://www.biomedcentral.com/bmcophthalmol/authors/instructions

    - *Eye News* (not listed on PubMed)
      http://www.eyenews.uk.com/contact-2

    - *Journal of Medical Case Reports* (requires payment)
      http://www.jmedicalcasereports.com/authors/instructions

    - *Journal of the Royal Society of Medicine*
      http://jrs.sagepub.com

- **Audit**

  Audit is now an important part of clinical practice. All doctors are expected to have an understanding of the audit process and to actively participate in it. Briefly, audit is the process of evaluating whether local practices match with a set standard. The set standard can be based on local / national guidelines or other published evidence. The analysis of any discrepancies should result in the implementation of a change in practice. A repeat audit in the future would ideally show an improvement in the local practice towards the level of the set standard, thereby completing the audit cycle.

  An audit that will impress shortlisters is one that:
  - *Is relevant to day-to-day clinical practice*
  - *Results in a change in practice for the better*
  - *Has been closed (i.e. improvement has been demonstrated)*

  To be involved in audit, make your interest known to your mentors and other consultant ophthalmologists. There are often areas that they have been unable to find the time to audit. You will need to set aside at least 6 months to complete an audit; it may be another 12 months before you can re-audit to complete the audit cycle.

  Top tips:
  - *Contact the ethics committee early.* If formal ethics approval is required, then start the process earlier rather than later. If the committee says that no formal ethics approval is needed, then you will have a written email / letter stating such. This is VERY useful when submitting your audit to journals for publication.

  - *Contact the audit department early* for assistance with patient identification, case notes retrieval, and data analysis.

  Potential quick audits with scope for improvement in practice include:
  - *Eyes in an A&E setting* – outcomes of eye emergencies
  - *Eyes in General Practice* – how referrals may be improved

21

- **Research**

  As mentioned earlier, the major issue with completing a piece of high quality research is time – a commodity which most FY doctors do not have. Generally, research takes at the very least 2 years from the start of the design process to actual acceptance of the manuscript by a peer-reviewed journal. Virtually all research involving NHS patients or staff would require some form of ethics input. As the ethics applications process can take up to 6 months, it is always best to contact the local ethics committee as early as possible for advice. The National Research Ethics Service (http://www.nres.nhs.uk) also provides useful information. Even though you may be unable to complete the research project in its entirety, it is still beneficial to be involved in the planning stages. Obtaining ethical approval in itself is viewed in good light as it demonstrates good planning, organisational and administrative skills. If you contribute sufficiently to data collection, data analysis or manuscript writing, you can then also meet the criteria for authorship of the eventual publication.

  To be involved in research, speak to your mentors as well as consultant ophthalmologists with an academic interest.

  Possibly the quickest route to publication (although that does not imply less hard work), may be these options:
  - *Cochrane reviews*
    http://www.cochrane.org/training/authors
    The Cochrane Collaboration aims to provide evidence for medical decision making by conducting systematic reviews for medical and surgical interventions. For ophthalmology, this is performed by the Cochrane Eyes & Vision Group (http://www.eyes.cochrane.org; CEVG). A good starting point would be to contact CEVG regarding the intervention you would like to perform a systematic review on. CEVG will then guide you on the workshops / courses that you will need to attend, as well as on the protocol and review preparation process.

- *Systematic literature reviews*

  Most peer-reviewed ophthalmology journals welcome systematic literature reviews on any particular topic. Unlike Cochrane reviews, these reviews do not have to focus solely on medical or surgical interventions. The reviews for these journals are also generally in a different format (dependent on the journal) to that required for a Cochrane review, and requires a broader search of the literature to include case series and case reports (if significant). After agreeing on a topic, you need to outline your review into several clear sections, e.g. Epidemiology, Genetics, Pathophysiology, Clinical Features, Investigations, Management and Prognosis. Once that has been done, email the Editor of any ophthalmology journal to put forward the case for the need to publish such a review. If the Editor agrees to it, then you'll need to write the article based on the journal requirements. The manuscript will still be subjected to the peer review process before it can be published. Although writing a systematic literature review does not require ethics approval, it still requires a substantial amount of time and effort. Dependent on the journal and the quality of the work, expect to have to review and summarise at least 50 to over 200 publications.

- *Questionnaire-based cross-sectional studies*

  There has been a proliferation of such studies looking at various topics ranging from departmental guidelines for the management of ocular diseases, clinician practice regarding certain procedures, junior training issues, and patient experience following different interventions. Please note that these studies generally require some form of ethical approval, and that the study may suffer from a poor response rate. Also, you will need to obtain some form of funding to cover the costs of printing and mailing out questionnaires and reminders.

- **Research Grants / Funding**

  An important issue to consider when conducting research is the issue of funding. Clearly, if possible, you would not want to have to spend money on top of all that extra work that you are already putting in. Research funding is usually obtained through a competitive process, and involves preparing a study protocol, completing an application form, justifying the effort of conducting the research, and outlining the projected costs required to fund the study until completion. Most research grant charities require evidence of formal ethical approval before funding is approved. Your supervisor will have some idea about where to apply for grants. Most NHS trusts have money set aside to fund research projects. In addition, some medical schools also provide small grants to ex-graduates. It is worth enquiring at the Research & Development department of your local hospital and the administrative office of your graduating medical school.

  External sources of financial support for research include:

  - *Medical Research Council Grants*
    http://www.mrc.ac.uk/Fundingopportunities/Grants/index.htm

  - *Guide Dogs UK Ophthalmic Research Grants*
    http://www.guidedogs.org.uk/aboutus/whatwedo/research/ophthalmic-research/#.UhF1a6y6-rs

  - *Chief Scientist Office Scotland Research Grants*
    http://www.cso.scot.nhs.uk/grants

  - *Tenovus Scotland*
    http://www.tenovus-scotland.org.uk/ForResearchers.html

  - *Ross Foundation for the Prevention of Blindness*
    http://www.s-o-c.org.uk/Grants-and-Bursaries.html

  - *Royal College of Surgeons of Edinburgh Ophthalmology Grants*
    http://www.rcsed.ac.uk/fellows-members/awards-and-grants/grants.aspx

Conducting research and audit can be a time-consuming and frustrating affair. Do persevere as it will be worth it in the long run. Here are some suggestions that you may find useful:

- **Collaborate with like-minded colleagues**

  Working with colleagues with similar interests will ease your burden and act as a source of motivation. Be sure to make clear who the main author will be right at the start to avoid disagreements later.

- **Pick a publishable topic**

  The last thing you want is to spend a lot of time on a dead-end project that no one wants to publish. Perform a literature search on PubMed (http://www.ncbi.nlm.nih.gov/pubmed) on the topics that you are considering. This will give you an idea of what has been done before and what you can potentially publish. Thereafter, it is important to discuss these potential topics with academically-minded ophthalmologists who will be able to tell you if the topics are publishable and worth your time. Finally, it is also crucial that you have some interest in the topic – nothing is worse than spending prolonged periods of time on something you have no enthusiasm for.

- **Plan ahead**

  Give yourself time. You will need at least 12 months from starting the project to having your manuscript eventually accepted for publication. Make sure you start the ethics application process as early as possible and commence your grant applications concurrently.

- **Set a framework and protocol**

  When you start your project, you need to know what you hope to achieve and how you will achieve it. After deciding on the aims of the study, you will need to ascertain the proper research methodology to achieve those aims. A statistician will be able to advise you on the data required and how the data should be analysed. Follow your planned protocol as closely as possible to minimise study bias.

- **Minimise data loss**

  Reduce your risk of incomplete data by preparing a data collection table. If yours is a prospective study, create a timetable for study participants to follow. Remind them of their scheduled appointments a few days beforehand. Enter the data into your database as soon as they become available. Remember to always back up your data!

- **Writing and submitting your scientific manuscript**

  In general, manuscripts are divided into the following sections:
  - *Introduction / Background*
  - *Aims / Purpose*
  - *Materials and Methods.* This should include a description of the statistical analysis methods and ethics approval status.
  - *Main Outcome Measures*
  - *Results.* Remember that it is unnecessary to replicate in text what you will be conveying in the results tables and graphs.
  - *Discussion and Conclusion.* This should include weaknesses of your study and the measures that were taken to mitigate them.
  - *References, Tables, Figures, Legend*

  Do not wait until all your data has been collected before you start writing your paper. In fact, start working on the introduction and methods as early as possible. Drawing up the results tables first may help in structuring your discussion. For basic statistical analysis, PSPP (http://www.gnu.org/software/pspp) can be useful. Consider using referencing software, such as Zotero (http://www.zotero.org), to organise your references. Obtain feedback first before submitting your manuscript, and be aware of the different submission guidelines (accessible from the journal websites) for the different journals. Submit your manuscript with a cover letter and a copyright transfer form signed by all authors. Journals usually reply within 3 months with comments from the reviewers. Don't despair if your manuscript is rejected; there are many other journals that you can re-submit to.

- **Ophthalmology journals**

  Listed below, in alphabetical order, is a selection of ophthalmology journals that you can submit your manuscripts to:

  - *Acta Ophthalmologica (formerly Acta Ophthalmologica Scandinavica)*
    http://onlinelibrary.wiley.com/journal/10.1111/%28ISSN%291755-3768/homepage/ForAuthors.html

  - *American Journal of Ophthalmology*
    http://www.ajo.com/authorinfo

  - *JAMA Ophthalmology (formerly Archives of Ophthalmology)*
    http://archopht.jamanetwork.com/public/InstructionsForAuthors.aspx

  - *British Journal of Ophthalmology*
    http://bjo.bmj.com/site/about/guidelines.xhtml

  - *Clinical & Experimental Ophthalmology*
    http://onlinelibrary.wiley.com/journal/10.1111/%28ISSN%291442-9071/homepage/ForAuthors.html

  - *Eye*
    http://mts-eye.nature.com/cgi-bin/main.plex?form_type=display_auth_instructions

  - *Graefe's Archive for Clinical & Experimental Ophthalmology*
    http://www.springer.com/medicine/ophthalmology/journal/417

  - *Investigative Ophthalmology & Visual Science*
    http://www.iovs.org/site/misc/author.xhtml

  - *Journal of Cataract & Refractive Surgery*
    http://www.elsevier.com/journals/journal-of-cataract-and-refractive-surgery/0886-3350/guide-for-authors

  - *Ophthalmology*
    http://www.aaojournal.org/authorinfo

Conferences / Congresses / Meetings

The obvious downside to attending conferences is that they are expensive, especially if you have no access to any study leave funds. The good news is that registration fees are usually discounted for students and trainees, and are tax deductible. Try to attend at least 2 meetings each year.

The benefits of attending conferences are numerous; much more so if you are presenting findings from studies that you have been involved in:

- Oral or poster presentation to disseminate research work
- Opportunity to practise presentation skills
- Opportunity to win prizes awarded for the best presentation / poster (this will look excellent on the CV)
- Opportunity to attend instructional courses or workshops
- Opportunity to travel and network

It can be easy to feel overawed when attending a meeting where you do not know anyone and even less about the topics that are being discussed. It can be difficult to strike up a conversation with a total stranger, even more so someone who is at a higher seniority level than you. However, most ophthalmologists are very friendly and approachable, and are often happy to talk to those wanting to start out. Create a good impression by dressing appropriately, and by being polite and concise. Do some reading beforehand so that when you do meet someone you can speak to, you are able to engage in a reasonable level of conversation. If your mentor or someone you know is also present at the same meeting, ask to be introduced to other ophthalmologists. Pay attention to presentations made by others – use that as a starting reference point for your encounter.

"Hello, I'm Amy Loid, FY2 in Edinburgh. I found your talk very interesting, particularly that discussion about ..."

If possible, obtain a contact email address so that you can send a follow-up "thank you" email soon after the meeting – this will help to reinforce the impression the ophthalmologists have of you.

These conferences can be at the local hospital, regional, national, and international levels. Below is a list of meetings that you can present at:

- **Regional and National**
    - *North of England Ophthalmological Society Meeting*
      http://www.neos.org.uk/html/meetings.html

    - *Oxford Ophthalmological Congress*
      http://www.oxford-ophthalmological-congress.org.uk/page.asp?node=55&sec=Conference

    - *Royal College of Ophthalmologists Annual Congress*
      http://www.rcophth.ac.uk/events.asp?eventfilter=0001300000020004&section=23&sectionTitle=Events

    - *Scottish Ophthalmology Club Meeting*
      http://www.s-o-c.org.uk/meetings.php

    - *South Western Ophthalmological Society Meeting*
      http://www.swos.org.uk/pages/article.asp?Sec=18

- **International**
    - *American Academy of Ophthalmology Annual Meeting*
      http://www.aao.org/meetings/annual_meeting

    - *Association for Research in Vision and Ophthalmology Meeting*
      http://www.arvo.org/Conferences_and_Courses

    - *Asia Pacific Academy of Ophthalmology Annual Congress*
      http://www.apaophth.org

    - *European Association for Vision & Eye Research Congress*
      http://www.ever.be/news.php

    - *Royal Australian & New Zealand College of Ophthalmologists Annual Scientific Congress*
      http://www.ranzco.edu/index.php/communications/events

It can be daunting when you present at a conference for the very first time. Don't worry; most ophthalmologists are friendly and very supportive of newcomers. Here are some suggestions that may help:

- **Conference presentation guidelines**

  These will be available from the conference website. The first priority is to submit your abstract before the abstract submission deadline. If you have a poster presentation, ensure that your poster conforms to the poster dimension guidelines. For oral presentations, make sure that yours does not exceed the allotted time (usually between 3 to 8 minutes with an additional 1 to 5 minutes for questions).

- **Start your preparations early**

  For poster presentations, contact the medical illustration department at your hospital or affiliated university at least 4 weeks in advance of the conference. This gives the department a chance to produce a poster, show it to you, and subsequently make changes to the poster based on your instructions. If you have a podium presentation, rehearse your talk as early as you can, ideally in front of colleagues who are able to provide constructive feedback. Whichever presentation type, you need to know your material inside out. Try to predict the questions that your audience may ask, and prepare your answers accordingly. Finally, make sure you submit your study leave application and make travel, visa and accommodation arrangements.

- **On the day of the presentation**

  Dress smartly. Put up your poster on the correct poster board and upload your presentation in advance. If you have embedded audio or video in your presentation, check that it works. Have a look around the stage that you'll be presenting at so that you have an idea of what it would be like when you are up there facing the audience. When it is your turn to present, speak clearly and do not rush. Finally, remember to thank your audience at the end of your presentation.

Examinations

Well, what is postgraduate life without the shadow of looming exams? Unfortunately, there is no running away from them, especially in a competitive field such as ophthalmology. OST trainees only need to sit for the FRCOphth Part 1 exam when already within the training programme. However, the reality is that many applicants would already have sat for (to varying degrees of success) an ophthalmology basic science exam prior to their OST application. The main drawbacks of sitting for basic science postgraduate exams are the cost and the stress of exam preparation.

However, there are 3 key benefits that outweigh the drawbacks:
- Demonstrates your commitment to a career in ophthalmology
- Improves your knowledge in ophthalmic basic sciences
- Passing is an impressive achievement that will make your CV glow

There are various exams that one can sit for. You need not limit yourself to taking only one exam. After all, the study content is the same and can be used interchangeably between exams. However, please note that *apart from the FRCOphth Part 1, the other College exams are not recognised for training purposes in the UK*, although they may offer advantages if you are considering practising abroad.

- **Royal College of Ophthalmologists FRCOphth Part 1**
  http://www.rcophth.ac.uk/page.asp?section=145&sectionTitle=Examination+Application+Packs

- **Royal College of Surgeons of Edinburgh FRCSEd(Ophth) Part A**
  http://www.rcsed.ac.uk/examinations/ophthalmology.aspx

- **Royal College of Physicians & Surgeons of Glasgow FRCS (Ophthalmology) Part 1**
  http://www.rcpsg.ac.uk/en/surgeons/examinations-and-assessment/frcs-ophthalmology/part-1.aspx

- **International Council of Ophthalmology (ICO) Basic Science Exam**
  http://www.icoexams.org/exams

Below are some suggestions to aid in your revision and preparations for the FRCOphth Part 1 basic science examinations:

- **Effective time management**

  Effective time management is crucial towards your success in the FRCOphth Part 1. Once you have decided to sit for the exam, you should begin your preparations at least 6 months beforehand. Try to allocate at least 2 hours per day for study, more during weekends.

- **Part 1 revision books**

  http://ophthalmologytraining.blogspot.com/p/related-books.html

  http://www.eyedocs.co.uk/ophthalmology-reviews/general/books
  - *Basic Sciences in Ophthalmology: A Self Assessment Test* by John Ferris
  - *Biochemistry of the Eye* by David Whikehart
  - *Clinical Anatomy of the Eye* by Richard Snell
  - *Clinical Optics* by Andrew Elkington
  - *Revision in Sciences Basic to Ophthalmology* by Raman Malhotra
  - *Study Guide for the FRCOphth* by Sunil Shah
  - *The Eye: Basic Sciences in Practice* by John Forrester
  - *Selection of revision books* by Marudi Publications

    http://www.mrcophth.com/marudi/marudipublications1.html

- **Part 1 revision courses and internet resources**
  - *Intensive Revision Course in Basic Sciences for Ophthalmic Exams*

    http://www.ucl.ac.uk/ioo-courses/frcop

  - *Success in MRCOphth*

    http://www.mrcophth.com

  - *Muthusamy Virtual University of Postgraduate Ophthalmology*

    http://www.mvupgo.com

Ophthalmology Courses / Workshops

Attending courses and workshops is one of the best ways of bolstering the CV without having to put in too much effort. It generally involves filling in an application form and then sending it to the course organisers along with an enclosed signed bank cheque or credit card details.

Although they can be expensive, attending these courses / workshops is advantageous in various ways:
- Improves the CV
- Imparts relevant and interesting knowledge on the subject matter
- Allows immediate clarification of ambiguous questions or issues
- Provides a good platform for networking with peers and seniors

The following is a list of some ophthalmology courses currently being run for current OST trainees as well as for those interested in taking up a career in ophthalmology. They are by no means endorsed by the authors nor are there any financial interests.

- **Basic Microsurgical Skills Course, Royal College of Ophthalmologists**
  http://www.rcophth.ac.uk/page.asp?section=681&sectionTitle=Microsurgical+Skills+Courses
  The Basic Microsurgical Skills Course focuses on the use of the operating microscope and handling of microsurgical instruments and ocular tissues. All OST trainees are required to attend the course as it is a prerequisite to performing any kind of ocular surgery.

- **Edinburgh FOCUS – Foundation Course in Ophthalmology**
  http://www.edinburgh-focus.com
  This is an introductory course designed to teach the basic practical skills required by new doctors working in ophthalmology and those wanting to learn basic ophthalmic examination skills.

- **Intensive Revision Course in Basic Sciences for Ophthalmic Exams**
  http://www.ucl.ac.uk/ioo-courses/frcop
  This revision course covers the topics examined for the FRCOphth Part 1 and ICO Basic Science assessments. The course includes theoretical optics and refraction as well as examination techniques.

- **Ophthalmology for GPs – Taking the fear out of ophthalmology**
  http://www.eyelearn.org.uk/course-gps.html
  This course covers the assessment and management of common paediatric and adult eye conditions. While it is aimed primarily at GPs, it should also be of benefit to any doctor interested in ophthalmology.

- **Tropical ophthalmology**
  http://www.lshtm.ac.uk/study/cpd/sto.html
  This 3-day course is aimed at ophthalmologists both in the United Kingdom and overseas wishing to gain more information on eye diseases found in the tropics.

This list is by no means exhaustive; so keep a watch out for other advertised courses, either over the internet or at your hospital eye department notice boards. Informative websites for courses include:
- http://www.eyelearn.org.uk
- http://www.rcophth.ac.uk/page.asp?section=315&sectionTitle=Curriculum+Based+Courses
- http://www.mkupdate.co.uk/courses.php
- http://www.moorfields.nhs.uk/Healthprofessionals/Medicaleducation/Ourcourses
- http://www.buos.co.uk/index.php/bevents/upcomingevents

Other Courses / Workshops

Although these courses are not directly related to ophthalmology, they do impart skills and knowledge that prospective employers and colleagues will all find attractive. This is particularly so if attending such courses enhances skills that complement those already present within the department. In this day and age, evidence is all important, so make sure you collect and keep your certificates of attendance or completion. It is no good saying that you can do this or that without being able to back up your claims.

Try to have something in your CV in each of the following broad categories:

- **Clinical**
  - *Advanced Life Support (ALS)*
    http://www.resus.org.uk/pages/alsinfo.htm
  - *Advanced Trauma Life Support (ATLS)*
    http://www.rcseng.ac.uk/courses/course-search/atls.html

- **Communication**
  - *Communication Skills Workshop for Foundation Doctors New to the NHS*
    http://www.londondeanery.ac.uk/professional-development/professional-support-unit/communication-skills/induction-and-communication-skills-workshop-for-foundation-doctors-new-to-the-nhs
  - *Communication Challenges in Hospital Practice*
    http://www.ec4h.org.uk/our-courses
  - *Hammersmith Communication Skills for Doctors*
    http://www.medicalcommunicationskills.com/communicationskillscourse.html
  - *Advanced Communication Skills for Doctors*
    http://www.medicalinterviewsuk.co.uk/advanced-communication-skills-course.html

- **Interview**
  - *Hammersmith Interview Skills for Doctors*
    http://www.medicalcommunicationskills.com/specialty_interviews.html

  - *Interview Skills for Junior Doctors*
    http://bma.org.uk/events/2013/tag/interview-skills-for-junior-doctors

  - *Oxford Medical ST Interview Course*
    http://www.medicalinterviewsuk.co.uk/st-interview-course.html

- **Presenting**
  - *Presenting and Influencing*
    http://bma.org.uk/events/tag/presenting-and-influencing

  - *Oxford Medical Presentation Skills Course*
    http://www.medicalinterviewsuk.co.uk/oxford-medical-courses/medical-presentation-skills/view-category.html

- **Management**
  - *Oxford Medical Essentials of Management and Leadership Course*
    http://www.medicalinterviewsuk.co.uk/1-day-management/leadership/essentials-of-medical-management-and-leadership/view-category.html

  - *Management Essentials*
    http://bma.org.uk/events/tag/management-essentials

- **Teaching**
  - *Effective Teaching Skills Workshop*
    http://www.rcplondon.ac.uk/cpd/non-clinical-cpd/teaching/effective-teaching-skills-workshop

  - *Teaching Skills 4 GPs*
    http://www.medicalskillscourses.com/teachingskills4GPs

- **Research & Statistics**
  - *Clinical Research Training for Scotland Courses*
    http://www.crts.org.uk/national/Courses.aspx

  - *Evidence-Based Practice Workshop*
    http://www.cebm.net/index.aspx?o=1732

  - *Learn Medical Statistics*
    http://www.learn-medical-statistics.com

  - *Medical Statistics for Non-Statisticians*
    http://www.rostrumtrainingsolutions.com/coursedetail.aspx?id=27

  - *Practical Statistics for Medical Research*
    http://www.ucl.ac.uk/stats/psmr

- **Information technology (IT)**
  - *IT User Qualifications (ITQ) Levels 1 and 2*
    http://www.learndirect.co.uk/qualifications/computers-it/itq/

  - *European Computer Driving Licence (ECDL)*
    http://www.ecdluk.co.uk

- **Courses run by medical organisations**
  - The *British Medical Association (BMA)*
    http://bma.org.uk/developing-your-career/foundation-training/bma-careers-elearning

  - The *Royal College of Surgeons of Edinburgh*
    http://www.rcsed.ac.uk/education/courses-and-events/foundation-trainees.aspx

  - The *Royal College of Physicians of London*
    http://www.rcplondon.ac.uk/cpd/non-clinical-cpd/teaching

  - The *Royal Society of Medicine (RSM)*
    http://www.rsm.ac.uk/academ/coursediary.php

Charity / Volunteer Work

"Every good act is charity. A man's true wealth hereafter is the good that he does in this world to his fellows." Moliere

One of the most rewarding aspects of ophthalmology is the impact it achieves in improving patients' vision and quality of life. In developed countries, the satisfaction from such successes can be somewhat diluted due to the hustle and bustle of regimented clinics and high expectations from patients and ophthalmologists alike. Charity work and volunteering abroad offers you the chance to step out of your comfort zone, and to appreciate the gift of sight at a more elementary level. It provides an opportunity to contribute where help is most needed, learn new skills, and experience different cultures. Being involved in charity work showcases a commitment to ophthalmology outside of the working environment, demonstrates planning and organisational skills, and promotes a sense of duty in community and global health care. These are all qualities that will help you stand out as a well-rounded candidate.

Every good act is charity. There are literally hundreds of ways that you can contribute. Any effort and contribution will be appreciated, no matter how little or how much time or money you contribute. Just bring along your enthusiasm and an open mind! Listed below are some examples of how you can contribute and at the same time build up your ophthalmology CV:

- **Social service work**
  Spend some time talking to blind or partially sighted people. Offer to help with their groceries or drive them for home or social visits. You'll be amazed at how much your time is appreciated.

- **Local eye charities**
  Helping local eye charities can be as simple as manning the cash machine and distributing flyers, or as complex as organising educational sessions and designing websites related to eye health. It really is up to you how you want to help out.

- **Fundraising**

  The cornerstone for all aid organisations is the raising of funds and donations to finance their operations. You can choose to take part in fundraisers, challenges or activities that have already been planned by the charities. Alternatively, you can organise your own events that could involve your would-be sponsors – this way, you can enjoy light-hearted (or serious!) activities and collect donations simultaneously.

  It is now increasingly popular to fundraise for a worthy cause by attempting (and hopefully completing) a personal challenge of sorts. If you opt to raise funds this way, here are some helpful tips:

  - *Begin as early as possible*
    The idea is not only to persuade people to open up their wallets (this can take time) but also to spread the awareness of the importance of the cause you are fundraising for. Implement a planned and resolute approach to your fundraising. Always have with you donation leaflets to show to potential sponsors.

  - *Make a list and start with people you know*
    Create a longlist of family, friends, colleagues and associates of your family, friends, neighbours and work colleagues. Be clear in your mind how to approach them and what you want to say to them. You can reduce your workload by recruiting close friends and family to help you out. You can also speak to managers who control budgets at your affiliated clubs or to colleagues in other businesses. Approach the boss and ask if you can tell sponsors that donations will be matched pound for pound by the business.

  - *Use the power of the internet – social networking websites*
    A good way to expand your donation pool is through Facebook (http://www.facebook.com) and other social networking websites. You can use this as a forum to keep your sponsors updated with your progress and also for them to give you feedback.

- *Use the power of the internet – online donation webpage*

  This is now very easy to set up. Most charities have websites that host toolkits to set up donation pages with secure internet payment. You can include this webpage in your donation forms and email invites. This is a very effective method to reach your mass targets. Online donation is usually preferred by potential sponsors as they are at liberty to find out more about the charity and donate in their own privacy.

- *Persistence and the personal touch*

  Meeting face to face with your sponsors makes it difficult for them to ignore your requests. Always have your donation form ready and be resolute with your promotion efforts. Even if you are unsuccessful at first, ask for their contact details and for permission to discuss again. Approach anyone and everyone – you might just receive support from the unlikeliest sources!

- *Value for money*

  Sponsors want to know how their hard-earned money will be spent. So have a confident reply (rather than a vague answer) ready. Statements like "*£300 restores sight to 10 people while £1500 provides 300 brand new glasses for children and adults.*" will highlight to sponsors the likely impact of their contributions.

- *Make donating easy for your sponsors*

  Ensure your personal and contact details are legible and already completed in your sponsorship forms. If any sponsor wants to pay upfront – accept it! Always have information leaflets and contact details at hand.

- *Collect the money and thank your sponsors personally*

  Once you have completed your end of the deal, politely remind your sponsors of the amount you have been promised. Tell them how it went and thank them personally. Remember to emphasise to your sponsors how worthwhile their contributions will be.

- **Being a volunteer overseas**

  If you want a full hands-on experience and an understanding of the complexities and realities of global health, then consider volunteering abroad. The major charity organisations have well set-up programmes overseas where you can work with local ophthalmologists, optometrists and ophthalmic nurses to facilitate comprehensive eye care for patients living in poverty.

  Caution: Offering your help overseas does not mean an all expenses paid cruise trip for you to turn up and feel good about yourself. You will be expected to pay for your travel, food and lodging. You will also have to prepare and organise everything yourself. Some are discouraged by this, but do bear in mind that non-profit humanitarian organisations are unable to afford luxuries for volunteers. The sooner you can prepare for your trip, the better. Give yourself at least 4 to 6 months.

  - *Deciding where to go*

    Ask previous volunteers about their experience overseas. Charity mailing lists and Facebook pages are often excellent sources of information. Find out about the different programmes and ask yourself what you can bring to the local programme. For example, the more rural programmes may not always offer surgical opportunities to inexperienced doctors.

    Do not worry if you have little or no ophthalmology experience; every little help is precious and you will learn plenty from just participating. Speak to the charity bodies and discuss with them the goals or objectives that you want to achieve during your volunteer trip.

  - *Fundraising*

    See above for advice on how to raise funds for your trip.

- *What to bring*
Just turning up with your sunglasses and good intentions is not enough. Materials such as spectacles, ophthalmic examination equipment and medicines are needed urgently to continue vital support for eye care locally. Liaise with the local team to find out the provisions that are most needed in that locale.

- *Donations – medicines and ophthalmic examination equipment*
Opticians and optometrists are good sources of unwanted Snellen vision charts, eye occluders, pinholes, pen torches and so on. You can also try contacting hospital eye clinics to see if they have unutilised clinical equipment available for donation. Speak to ophthalmic pharmaceutical representatives for sample eye drops and medications which you can bring overseas.

- *Donations – spectacles*
Many optical and optometry businesses collect old unwanted glasses from their customers for distribution to charity bodies. You can approach your local opticians and optometrists for these spectacles. Most will be more than happy to oblige as this helps to clear out their store rooms at the same time.

One tip is to ask them about their affiliated charities and collection depots for donated spectacles. You will be able to obtain a greater number of glasses this way and save valuable time in the process.

In the UK, Vision Aid (see below) provides an excellent source of donated spectacles. Contact them about your volunteer project and enquire if they can provide you with supplies.

- **Travel considerations**
  - Plan early and ensure that you fulfil all visa requirements
  - Get international medical and security insurance
  - Inform the overseas programme organiser of your emergency contact information and flight itinerary
  - Leave the contact details of the local organiser and your lodging place with your family so that they know how to reach you
  - Register with your embassy at the foreign destination
  - Be up-to-date with your vaccinations – consult the following websites for travel vaccination advice:
    - http://www.cdc.gov/travel
    - http://www.netdoctor.co.uk/travel/vaccines_index.shtml
    - http://www.nhs.uk/conditions/travel-immunisation/Pages/Introduction.aspx
  - Leave a copy of your passport at home with a family member
  - Predict financial needs: bring local currency and find out about ATM / currency exchange facilities in the area where you will be
  - Bring adapters for electrical items
  - Sunscreen, insect repellent, first aid supplies and a free-standing mosquito net would not go amiss either!

- **Other helpful tips**
  - Find out the local customs and be sensitive about respecting and observing cultural norms
  - Go into this exciting experience with an open mind and try to immerse yourself in the local culture. Flexibility allows for a more enjoyable and rewarding experience in a foreign country.
  - Make time to really get to know people, from your local team members to the patients and their relatives
  - Do not be afraid to ask questions or to strike up a conversation with the local team members. The more effort you put into the experience, the easier it is for them to teach you.
  - Keep a log or journal about your experiences

- **Suggested Eye Charities**

  For volunteering abroad, organisations like Unite for Sight, Vision Aid and ORBIS have very well set-up programmes overseas. They are all very approachable and will always be happy to provide assistance and advice to inexperienced starters.

  - *Unite For Sight*

    http://www.uniteforsight.org

    This international volunteer organisation encourages undergraduate, public health, medical, and graduate students to engage in front-line service programmes in deprived areas throughout the world. Unite For Sight provides excellent guidance as well as online training modules for volunteers intending to participate in any of the service programmes.

  - *ORBIS*

    http://www.orbis.org

    ORBIS is global development organisation providing long-term capacity projects and eye care in places like Bangladesh and Ethiopia. It is famed for conducting eye surgery aboard custom-designed aeroplanes. ORBIS can help you plan fundraising events while at the same time raising awareness of their sight-saving work worldwide. However, please note that ORBIS has stringent credentialing requirements and is quite selective about who can be involved as a medical volunteer.

  - *Vision Aid*

    http://www.vao.org.uk

    Vision Aid is an international eye charity organisation that conducts a variety of fundraisers in the UK and offers a broad opportunity to volunteer other countries, such as in India and Africa. It provides very helpful advice and support in organising your own fundraising events. It is also an excellent source of donated spectacles.

For those who do not have the inspiration or time to volunteer abroad, there are still plenty of opportunities to contribute locally. All charities, whether local or national, will be keen to hear from prospective volunteers. As previously mentioned, there are many ways to be involved – you can participate in planned charity events, or you can offer your skills and experience. Below are some well-known UK-based eye charity organisations that you may wish to contact:

- *Royal National Institute of Blind People (RNIB)*
  http://www.rnib.org.uk
  RNIB is a leading UK charity that aims to eliminate avoidable sight loss through the dissemination of information and campaigns. It also offers practical support and advice to people affected by sight loss. RNIB has information on a wide variety of local community volunteer programmes and activities in the United Kingdom.

- *Fight for Sight*
  http://www.fightforsight.org.uk
  Fight for Sight is the leading charity organisation in the UK dedicated to funding research into the prevention and treatment of blindness and eye diseases. It offers a selection of fundraiser events as well as opportunities for supporting ophthalmic-related research.

- *Sightsavers International*
  http://www.sightsavers.org
  Sightsavers International is a UK-based charity that aims to reduce blindness in developing countries through specialist treatment and eye care. For those who are already blind, Sightsavers International provides education, counselling and training. It organises a variety of events to raise vital funds for its programmes abroad.

Other Contributions

If after all this, you still find that you have some spare time in your hands (!), then there are yet more things that you can do to gain those extra brownie points. Anything that contributes toward the local ophthalmology department in any manner will be viewed positively. Realistically, the main areas where your contributions would most likely be appreciated would be in relation to teaching and to the organisation of events / sessions.

- **Journal club**

    Attending journal club sessions increases your exposure to the recent advances in ophthalmology. Some topics may initially be too advanced for someone new to ophthalmology, so it may be better for you to pick and choose the sessions to attend. You may even want to summarise and present some articles at these sessions. Start by choosing a reasonably simple eye-related publication which you find interesting. Preparing for journal club meetings will help you build up your critical analysis and presentation skills in a fairly friendly and non-confrontational setting. If there are no journal club sessions, why not speak to your mentors or one of the consultant ophthalmologists and offer to organise such sessions on a weekly or fortnightly basis?

- **Departmental teaching sessions**

    Most units will have a weekly departmental teaching session. Find out when they are from the department secretary, and try to attend some of these sessions. Let your mentors or a consultant ophthalmologist know of your interest in attending. Better yet, offer to present an interesting case or two at some of these sessions. Give yourself at least one week to prepare the case presentations. It is usually instructive to go through the case with someone else first to iron out any problems before the actual presentation itself. Do not get disheartened if you feel that your presentation did not go well; you would often have performed much better than you think.

- **Medical student teaching**

  The teaching of medical students is often delegated to the trainee. In addition, there is often insufficient structured ophthalmology teaching for medical students. If there are any aspects of medical student teaching that can be improved upon, then it may be worthwhile contacting the consultant ophthalmologist in charge of student teaching to volunteer your help in rectifying the deficient areas. For instance, if the medical students are not receiving enough clinical skills teaching, then offer to organise formal lunchtime teaching sessions or tutorials at the end of the clinic. Most ophthalmologists will be delighted to support to such efforts.

- **Computer assisted learning packages / Podcasts**

  The education of medical students is not limited to direct face-to-face teaching. Most universities now have computer assisted learning packages and podcasts on various aspects of medicine. To set these up would involve speaking to the ophthalmology department as well as the relevant university department. With the blessings of your mentors and consultant ophthalmologists, pick a few common or important ocular conditions (for instance, acute primary angle closure, ocular chemical injury, optic neuritis, endophthalmitis, etc) and offer to set up a computer assisted learning package / podcast for medical students. Instead of doing everything yourself, it may be better to share out the workload among similarly inclined colleagues.

- **Local protocols / guidelines**

  You can also contribute to the drafting of local protocols. Speak to your mentors or any of the local consultants to see if there are any aspects of local practice that require guidelines. The purpose of the guidelines may be to standardise patient care or to streamline services. Possible topics include the management of acute primary angle closure, the management of orbital cellulitis, the cataract care pathway and the referral process for out-of-hours eye casualty.

- **Extracurricular activities**

    You may wish to involve yourself in activities outside of the hospital and university setting. Demonstrating talent and success in extracurricular activities, such as in sport or music adds to what makes you unique and gives the interview panel an insight into another facet of your personality. In addition, it shows that you are an all-rounded character with other interests besides ophthalmology. If you are accomplished in something, make sure the shortlisting and interview panels know about it – highlight it in your CV, emphasise it in your application forms, and mention it during your interviews. Having common interests helps to break the ice and may well be the deciding factor that clinches you the job during your interview.

    Any voluntary work, even if not with eye-related charities, is seen in a positive light. You can involve yourself with organisations such as:

    - *British Red Cross*
        http://www.redcross.org.uk

    - *Médecins Sans Frontières*
        http://www.msf.org.uk

    - *Samaritans*
        http://www.samaritans.org

    - *St John Ambulance*
        http://www.sja.org.uk/sja/default.aspx

    If you are able to converse in different languages, you may wish to consider volunteering as a clinical interpreter at your local hospital. Remember that voluntary work is not limited only to large organisations or the hospital – you can easily volunteer to help at a day care centre for disabled children or at a homeless shelter. Contributing to society is immensely satisfying, and at the same time you'll be further developing useful skills, such as people and time management, negotiation, and communication skills.

- **Website contribution**

One of the best ways of disseminating educational information and material about eye health and eye care to the public is via the internet. Independent information websites, such as Vision & Eye Health (http://www.vision-and-eye-health.com), as well as charity information and online news websites, often welcome contributions from external sources. If you are keen to write articles about eye conditions with important public health implications (e.g. blindness from glaucoma) for such websites, then it is worthwhile contacting the webmaster to find out how you can contribute. Most webmasters are happy to be approached by potential contributors. Writing such articles will improve your knowledge and your CV, and also raise your online public profile.

Writing public awareness articles is not the only way that you can contribute. If you have web design skills, you may be able to help a local charity or charities set up and design a website to raise their online profile. If you have the time, you can also help these charities maintain an online presence through social media. Contributing this way benefits both the charities and the local people that they serve.

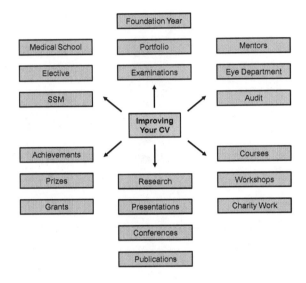

Figure 2: Summary of ways to improve your CV for OST applications

Chapter 3

The Applications Process

Shi Zhuan Tan

Brian Ang

The Applications Process

Ophthalmology Specialty Training:

Ophthalmology is a very competitive specialty. In 2013, there were 323 applications for 86 OST1 posts and no unfilled positions after Round 1 (http://www.severndeanery.nhs.uk/recruitment/vacancies/show/RCOphth-2/competition-ratios-lib). The competition was perhaps even tougher in previous years, with up to 89 applicants per post in 2010.

Recruitment into OST now occurs through a nationally coordinated process, in contrast to previously when it was conducted by the local Postgraduate Deaneries. Round 1 of the national application for OST posts open in November, while Round 2 starts in February. The actual OST1 job starts in August. The Royal College of Ophthalmologists provides guidance (http://www.rcophth.ac.uk/page.asp?section=616&sectionTitle=National+Recru itment+for+Ophthalmic+Specialist+Training) on OST applications. Up-to-date details on recruitment can be found in the MMC website:
http://www.mmc.nhs.uk/colleges__deaneries.aspx

Academic Clinical Fellowship:

For those who are interested in an academic career, there is the option of getting an Academic Clinical Fellowship (ACF) as a Year 1 Academic Specialty Trainee in Ophthalmology, also through a national recruitment process. There are around 15 ACF posts nationally (although this can change as the academic programmes change).

Applications open in October (a month before OST applications), and the process is generally the same as for OST applications. However, the application form and interview questions focus more on academic / research achievements, with greater exploration of your interest in an academic career in ophthalmology. For further details, please visit the National Institute for Health Research (NIHR) website:
http://www.nihrtcc.nhs.uk/intetacatrain/acfs

To maintain the fairness and transparency of the applications process, the national recruitment for OST must meet the minimum national standards:

- All posts must be advertised for a minimum of 4 weeks
- Advertisements, information for applicants, and application forms must be clearly structured so that:
  - They are accessible, particularly for applicants with disabilities
  - Relevant details are easily found when carrying out a search
- All applications must be made electronically
- Application forms and interviews must map to person specifications
- The nationally application form must be used
- Applicants can apply for as many training programmes as they wish
- Random recruitment and selection processes must not be used
- All applications submitted before the deadline must be considered
- Shortlisters and interviewers must not have access to the equal opportunities information or personal data
- Interviewers must take account of applicants' portfolios, application forms, structured CV and summary of their portfolio of evidence
- Applicants should be asked to bring their portfolios to the interview

When you are applying for OST or ACF, you will need to observe most, if not all, the following processes:

- Understanding the timeline
- Immigration criteria
- Portfolio preparation
- Information gathering: Person specification
- Information gathering: Postgraduate Deanery
- Referees
- Application forms
- Shortlisting
- Interviews
- Offers
- The next step

Timeline

Ophthalmology Specialty Training Timeline

- *November:*   Start of Round 1 OST applications
- *December:*   Closing date for Round 1 OST applications
- *December – January:*   Eligibility checks and shortlisting
- *January – February:*   Invitation for interview
- *February – March:*   Offers issued

- *February – March:*   Start of Round 2 OST applications
- *March:*   Closing date for Round 2 OST applications
- *April – May:*   Invitation for interview
- *May:*   Offers issued

- *August:*   Commence OST post

Academic Clinical Fellowship Timeline

- *October:*   Start of ACF applications
- *November:*   Closing date for ACF applications
- *November:*   Eligibility checks and shortlisting
- *December – January:*   Invitation for interview
- *January – February:*   Offers issued

- *August:*   Commence ACF post

Before you start, you need to know the timeline of the whole applications process – when the opening and closing dates are, and when the interview dates are if shortlisted. Make sure you are available during these times.

Plan your time well so that you are able to work on the application form, obtain feedback on it, and submit **with time to spare**. Late applications received after the closing date will not be accepted.

Finally, do not think that you can easily sneak into an OST programme in Round 2. Most of the time, all posts would already have been filled in Round 1, so there would no longer be any posts available in Round 2.

Immigration Considerations

Before you begin, you must ask yourself: "Do I have the right to work in the UK?" If you are a UK citizen or an European Economic Area (EEA) national or if you have been granted with an Indefinite Leave to Remain (permanent residence) visa, then you have the right to work in the UK.

However, if you are not any of the above, then you must assess your eligibility to work in the UK before even thinking about starting the applications process. You can apply for an OST post if you have:

- Dependent status, and no restriction as a doctor in training

- A Tier 1 visa and no restriction against working as a doctor in training
  http://www.ukba.homeoffice.gov.uk/visas-immigration/working/tier1/general

- A current Tier 2 visa and will continue training with the same sponsor
  http://www.ukba.homeoffice.gov.uk/visas-immigration/working/tier2/general

- A current Tier 4 visa for your Foundation training programme and continuous immigration status in the UK since graduating from a UK medical school, and you will be applying for a Tier 2 visa.
  http://www.ukba.homeoffice.gov.uk/visas-immigration/studying/adult-students

If you fulfil any of the visa conditions above, make sure you submit copies of the following documents (along with your application) as evidence of your immigration eligibility to work in the UK:

- Biometric residence card
- Date stamped passport
- Accompanying visa grant letter from the UK Home Office

Please visit the UK Border Agency website for more about work visas:
http://www.ukba.homeoffice.gov.uk/visas-immigration/working/comparisons

Portfolio: Foundation Year Training

http://www.foundationprogramme.nhs.uk/pages/home/training-and-assessment

The portfolio is an important way for the trainee to document the achievement of required learning outcomes and competencies during the course of his or her training thus far. Upon achievement of the Foundation learning outcomes and competencies, and successful completion of your Foundation training programme, you will be awarded a **Foundation Achievement of Competence Document (FACD) 5.2**. If you have completed a Foundation training programme within 3 years of applying, make sure you attach a copy of your FACD 5.2 certificate to your application.

If you are a current Foundation trainee, you will not yet have the FACD 5.2 certificate before you apply. This is ok as long as you obtain an FACD 5.2 certificate before you start your OST1 post in August. However, there is nothing to stop you from completing all the requisite learning outcomes for Foundation Year doctors and to have all the documentation on file before you apply. Be prepared to show your portfolio if asked during the interview. Make sure your portfolio contains only your own original work and that there are no patient identifiable data.

The Foundation Year learning outcomes, their codes, and how they are assessed are listed as follows:

- **Intravenous cannulation: Perform venesection, cannulation and set-up intravenous infusions**
  - Code: Practical Skills PS4
  - Assessment: Direct Observation of Procedural Skills

- **Blood culture: Take samples for blood culture**
  - Code: Practical Skills PS20
  - Assessment: Direct Observation of Procedural Skills

- **Hand hygiene: Perform the correct hand hygiene technique**
  - Code: Practical Skills PS21
  - Assessment: Trust-based accreditation; Multi-Source Feedback

- **Appraisal: Engaged in appraisal and revalidation**
  - Code: Attitudes, Ethics, Responsibilities AER9
  - Assessment: Record of discussion in portfolio

- **Probity: Aware of issues of probity and possible conflict of interest in professional practice**
  - Code: Attitudes, Ethics, Responsibilities AER11
  - Assessment: Statement in portfolio

- **Legal: All doctors must practise according to the GMC document Duties of a Doctor**
  - Code: Attitudes, Ethics, Responsibilities AER12
  - Assessment: Record of discussion in portfolio

- **Data Protection: Application of the law in relation to data protection and its relevance to health care**
  - Code: Attitudes, Ethics, Responsibilities AER13
  - Assessment: Record of discussion in portfolio

- **Human Tissue: Application of the law in relation to human tissue**
  - Code: Attitudes, Ethics, Responsibilities AER14
  - Assessment: Record of discussion in portfolio

- **Child Protection: Understands the roles and responsibilities of an ophthalmologist in child protection**
  - Code: Attitudes, Ethics, Responsibilities AER15
  - Assessment: Record of discussion in portfolio

- **Personal Health: Takes responsibility for the implications of personal health on professional practice**
  - Code: Continuing Professional Development CPD7
  - Assessment: Record of discussion in portfolio

If you have not been in and are not in a Foundation training programme, you will not receive an FACD 5.2 certificate. However, even if you are an international medical graduate not working in the UK, you can still apply for OST1 posts provided the following criteria are fulfilled:

- **Alternative Certificates**

  You will need to ask your supervising consultant to confirm your achievement of foundation competencies via Alternative Certificates, which are another way of providing evidence of competence for those who have not undergone Foundation training.

  There are 3 types of Alternative Certificates:
  - *Alternative Certificate A*: posts with acute medical responsibilities
  - *Alternative Certificate B*: posts without acute medical responsibilities
  - *Research Certificate*: established research post (MD or PhD)

  For the Alternative Certificates to be valid, they must be:
  - *Fully completed and signed by your supervising consultant*, who need not witness every competence, but should judge based on observation of your work and evidence you provide.
  - *Current*. Certificates differ yearly, so you cannot use previous years' certificates. The certificates for 2013 are found below:
    http://www.mmc.nhs.uk/specialty_training_2010/specialty_training_2 012/recruitment_process/stage_3_- _vacancies__applicat/certificates_a_and_b_for_f2_co.aspx
  - *Specific for each post*. If you have had 2 different posts, then you will need 2 different certificates. Posts must be of at least 3 months' duration (whole time equivalent), have been completed by the time you apply, and have been undertaken within 3 years of the start of OST (usually in August).

It is in your best interests to start compiling and completing all the requisite learning outcomes for FY doctors as early as possible. Have all the documentation ready and let your supervisor know in advance that you require Alternative Certificates to be completed.

- **Work experience**

  You must confirm that you have a minimum **24 months working experience**, either in the UK or overseas, since graduating from medical school. This can be a combination of:

  - 12 months satisfactory completion of a pre-registration, internship of FY1 post; and:

  - 12 months full time satisfactory completion in posts approved for the purposes of medical education by the relevant authority; or

  - 12 months full time experience at a publicly funded hospital in at least 2 specialties; or

  - 12 months full time FY2 position

  The following are not accepted as evidence of experience:
  - Clinical attachments
  - Higher professional examinations

If there are areas that you are uncertain about, make sure you contact the relevant Postgraduate Deanery for clarification particularly since conditions and criteria for applications can change on a yearly basis. You do not want to spend significant amounts of time gathering all the relevant paperwork only to find out that your application was rejected or delayed due to a technical discrepancy as a result of not following the latest guidelines.

Portfolio: Ophthalmology Specialty Training

http://curriculum.rcophth.ac.uk/assessments/portfolio

If you want to shine, you can consider working on some learning outcomes for OST1, but you will likely have to repeat them upon entry into OST1.

- **Corneal Foreign Body: Remove ocular surface foreign bodies**
  - Code: Practical Skills PS11
  - Assessment: Direct Observation of Procedural Skills

- **Ocular Irrigation: Carry out irrigation and ocular debridement**
  - Code: Practical Skills PS22
  - Assessment: Direct Observation of Procedural Skills

- **Microscope: Use the operating microscope**
  - Code: Surgical Skills SS2
  - Assessment: Objective Assessment of Surgical & Technical Skills

- **Aseptic Technique: Use aseptic surgical technique**
  - Code: Surgical Skills SS3
  - Assessment: Objective Assessment of Surgical & Technical Skills

- **Contagion: Prevent contagion and cross infection**
  - Code: Health Promotion / Disease Prevention HPDP2
  - Assessment: Trust-based training certificates

- **Body Language: Aware of importance of non-verbal communication**
  - Code: Communication C8
  - Assessment: Personal reflection; Multi-Source Feedback

- **Complaints: Respond appropriately to complaints**
  - Code: Communication C9
  - Assessment: Multi-Source Feedback

- **Professionals: Communicate effectively with others**
  - Code: Communication C10
  - Assessment: Multi-Source Feedback

- **Leave: Adequate communication to ensure efficient service provision with respect to planned and unplanned leave and on-call work**
  - Code: Communication C14
  - Assessment: Multi-Source Feedback

- **Portfolio: Maintain a personal portfolio**
  - Code: Information Handling IH4
  - Assessment: Portfolio

- **Information Technology: Use appropriate IT and email facilities**
  - Code: Information Handling IH5
  - Assessment: Portfolio

- **Good Medical Practice (GMP): Understands and applies the principles in the GMC document "Good Medical Practice"**
  - Code: Role in Health Service HS3
  - Assessment: Portfolio

- **Reflects: Adopts reflective practice**
  - Code: Continuing Professional Development CPD1
  - Assessment: Case-based Discussion; Portfolio

- **Limits: Aware of the limits of his / her own knowledge and insight into his / her own difficulty in understanding complex interactions**
  - Code: Continuing Professional Development CPD2
  - Assessment: Case-based Discussion; Portfolio

- **Self-Learning: Able to direct his / her own self-learning**
  - Code: Continuing Professional Development CPD3
  - Assessment: Portfolio

- **CPD: Participates in continued professional development**
  - Code: Continuing Professional Development CPD5
  - Assessment: Portfolio

Person Specification: Essential Criteria

Before submitting your OST application, you must look at the person specification to make sure that you fulfil all *essential* criteria. You are extremely unlikely to be successful in your application if you lack in any one of the essential criteria. The essential criteria in the 2013 person specification for OST1 applications were:

http://www.mmc.nhs.uk/pdf/PS%202013%20ST1%20Ophthalmology2.pdf

- **Qualifications**
  - MBBS or equivalent medical qualification

- **Eligibility**
  - Eligible to work in the UK
  - Eligible for full registration with the General Medical Council
  - Holds a current licence to practice
  - Minimum 2 years postgraduate medical experience by August
  - Evidence of current employment in a UK Foundation Programme Office (UKFPO) affiliated Foundation Programme
  - Not previously released from an OST programme

- **Fitness to practise**
  - Up to date and fit to practise safely

- **Language skills**
  - Able to communicate effectively in English (undergraduate medical training in English or IELTS score of at least 7 within past 24 months)

- **Health**
  - Meets professional health requirements in line with General Medical Council standards and Good Medical Practice

- **Career progression**
  - Able to provide a complete employment history
  - Career progression consistent with personal circumstances
  - Present performance is commensurate with totality of training
  - ≤18 months Ophthalmology experience by the time of appointment

- **Application completion**
  - All sections of the application form completed fully as per guidelines

- **Clinical knowledge & expertise**
  - Appropriate knowledge base and capacity to apply sound clinical judgement

- **Research skills**
  - Demonstrates understanding of the principles of research

- **Audit**
  - Evidence of active participation in audit

- **Personal skills**
  - Capacity to take in others' perspectives, sees patients as people, and able to develop rapport
  - Capacity to adapt language as appropriate to the situation; open and non-defensive
  - Capacity to work cooperatively with others and show leadership / authority where appropriate
  - Capacity to use logical / lateral thinking to solve problems and make decisions
  - Capacity to operate under pressure. Demonstrates initiative and resilience to cope with setbacks and adapt to rapidly changing circumstances.
  - Capacity to manage time and information effectively, as well as to prioritise clinical tasks

- **Probity**
  - Capacity to take responsibility for own actions. Demonstrates a non-judgemental approach towards others

- **Commitment to specialty**
  - Realistic insight into specialty. Demonstrates self-awareness and commitment to personal and professional development

This list may seem long and tedious to read (previous lists have been much longer), but you will do well to go through it and to make sure that you can show evidence of fulfilling every single one of these essential criteria. You do not want to spend a lot of time and effort preparing your CV and application, only to fail in the applications process because of a minor oversight and you end up having to wait another year before applying again.

This can and does happen. So make sure you check and double check your application before submission. In the 2013 applications, 5% (17 applications out of 323 applications) failed to progress through the initial check (http://www.severndeanery.nhs.uk/recruitment/vacancies/show/RCOphth-2/competition-ratios-lib). You do not want to be among this 5% who did not even get past the initial check of the application process when it is your turn to apply for an OST post.

If there are areas that you are uncertain about, such as your eligibility to work in the UK, English language standards or portfolio requirements, make sure you contact the relevant Postgraduate Deanery for clarification.

Person Specification: Desirable Criteria

Before you are even considered for shortlisting for the interview, you (along with every other applicant for OST posts) will have to fulfil all the essential criteria. Merely possessing all the essential criteria is not really sufficient for you to be shortlisted because everyone else also has them.

Hence, the crucial factor that determines how much you stand out is whether or not you possess any *desirable* criteria. The more desirable criteria you have, the better. If you can, make sure your CV does not have any gaps in these areas. In the 2013 person specification for OST1 applications, the desirable criteria were:

http://www.mmc.nhs.uk/pdf/PS%202013%20ST1%20Ophthalmology2.pdf

- **Clinical skills**
  - Shows aptitude for practical skills, e.g. hand-eye coordination and dexterity

- **Research skills**
  - Evidence of academic and research achievements, e.g. degrees, prizes, awards, distinctions, publications, presentations, etc.

- **Teaching**
  - Evidence of interest and experience in teaching

- **Commitment to specialty**
  - Attendance at training courses specific to ophthalmology
  - Activities / achievements relevant to ophthalmology

Below are additional desirable criteria in the 2012 person specification (http://www.mmc.nhs.uk/pdf/PS%202012%20CT1%20CST2.pdf) for OST1 applications that have not been included in the 2013 person specification:

- **Clinical skills**
  - Attendance at relevant courses, e.g. ALS, ATLS or equivalent

- **Academic / Research skills**
  - Evidence of participation in risk management or research

Postgraduate Deaneries

It is important to find out about the OST posts in the respective Postgraduate Deaneries before deciding on which region or city you want to spend the next 7 years of your life in. It is a good idea to speak to those already currently in post to find out more about the job itself, the work environment, learning and research opportunities, support from senior staff and allied health professionals, as well as work-life balance.

Listed below are the Postgraduate Deaneries in the UK offering OST posts. There are around 13 Postgraduate Deaneries in England, while Scotland, Northern Island and Wales are considered as one Postgraduate Deanery each. In the application form, you will be asked to rank your order of preference for Postgraduate Deanery locations. More information on this can be found on the Severn Deanery website:

http://www.severndeanery.nhs.uk/recruitment/vacancies/show/RCOphth

- **Scotland**

    http://www.nes.scot.nhs.uk/education-and-training/by-discipline/medicine.aspx

    The NHS Education for Scotland website provides information on OST in all the 4 Scottish deaneries:
    - *East of Scotland Deanery* (Dundee)
    - *North of Scotland Deanery* (Aberdeen)
    - *South East Scotland Deanery* (Edinburgh)
    - *West of Scotland Deanery* (Glasgow)

- **Wales**
    - *Wales Deanery* (Cardiff)
        http://www.walesdeanery.org/index.php/en/ophthalmology.html

- **Northern Ireland**
    - *Northern Ireland Deanery* (Belfast)
        http://www.nimdta.gov.uk/specialty-training/specialty-schools/surgery/surgical-specialties

- **England**
  - *East Midlands Deanery* (Nottingham)
    http://www.eastmidlandsdeanery.nhs.uk/page.php?id=998
  - *East of England Deanery* (Cambridge)
    http://www.eoedeanery.nhs.uk/medical/page.php?area_id=21
  - *Kent, Surrey and Sussex Deanery* (Maidstone & Surrey)
    http://kssdeanery.org/ophthalmology
  - *London Deanery* (London)
    http://www.londondeanery.ac.uk/specialty-schools/ophthalmology
  - *Mersey Deanery* (Liverpool)
    http://www.merseydeanery.nhs.uk/ophthalmology
  - *North Western Deanery* (Manchester)
    http://www.nwpgmd.nhs.uk/node/568
  - *Northern Deanery* (Newcastle)
    http://www.northerndeanery.nhs.uk/NorthernDeanery/specialty-training/ophthalmology
  - *Oxford Deanery* (Oxford)
    http://www.oxforddeanery.nhs.uk/specialty_schools/oxford_school_of_surgery/ophthalmology.aspx
  - *Peninsula Deanery* (Exeter & Plymouth)
    http://www.peninsuladeanery.nhs.uk/index.php?option=com_content&view=article&id=737&Itemid=832
  - *Severn Deanery* (Bristol)
    http://ophthalmology.severndeanery.org
  - *Wessex Deanery* (Southampton)
    http://www.wessexdeanery.nhs.uk/recruitment__careers/core__specialty_recruitment.aspx
  - *West Midlands Deanery* (Birmingham)
    http://www.westmidlandsdeanery.nhs.uk/SpecialtySchools/Ophthalmology.aspx
  - *Yorkshire and the Humber Deanery* (Leeds & Sheffield)
    http://www.yorksandhumberdeanery.nhs.uk/ophthalmology

Referees

You need referees to give you references to support your OST application. By now you should have a pretty good idea of who you would like to name as your referees supporting your application. Your referees need to have supervised an aspect of your clinical training **within the past 2 years**. These can be:

- Your mentor
- The consultant ophthalmologists whom you are currently working with or have worked with previously
- Your Special Studies Module supervisor
- Your elective supervisor
- Your research supervisor
- If you have taken a career break and do not have any referees from within the past 2 years, then you must include your 2 most recent supervisors

Contact your potential referees as early as possible to confirm that they are willing to be your referee and to support your OST application with a reference. Give them plenty of notice of when they will likely be required to do so. Better still, confirm with them their availability to be contacted to provide the reference within the application timeframe.

In the application form, make sure you include the following referee details:

- Name
- Position
- Address
- Current work telephone number
- Up-to-date work email address

If you are successful and are offered an OST post, but no references have been received, then you will not be issued a contract by your prospective employer.

Application Form

The national application form is completed online and submitted electronically. Being an online process, there may be initial technical difficulties, so it is better to register and start the process earlier rather than later. The application forms can change, so you may find significant differences with previous years' forms.

You only get *around 3 weeks* to complete the application form, so plan your time well. Keep your answers concise, honest and truthful. At the same time, do NOT be afraid to sell yourself well since nobody else will. Relate your answers to best patient care and patients' best interests. Stick to the maximum word count allowed, and correct all grammatical or spelling errors. Avoid using upper case as it is difficult to read. Finally, ask your mentors to review your application and to provide constructive feedback.

In the application form, there will be standard questions to assess your portfolio and your fulfilment of the essential and desirable person specifications. In general, there will be information-based and competency-based questions on the following:

- **Achievements within medicine**
  These include undergraduate and postgraduate degrees or qualifications, prizes, awards, distinctions.

- **Achievements outside medicine**
  Be sure to include any achievements in sports, music, writing, charity work, etc. as these show how well-rounded you are as an individual.

- **Employment history and experience in ophthalmology**
  Include all ophthalmology experience in the UK and outside the UK. Make sure you are able to provide evidence for any career gaps.

- **Interest and commitment towards ophthalmology**
  In this section, write about courses attended (the Basic Microsurgical Skills Course is almost compulsory nowadays), taster week, elective, SSMs, ophthalmology-related skills, etc.

- **Research**

  This is partly assessed by the number of publications in peer-reviewed journals. The level of involvement is important. It looks better if you were the one who designed and conducted the study.

- **Audit**

  Audit experience is expected of applicants and there will be one question on audit and whether or not the audit loop was closed.

- **Presentations**

  These may be poster, e-poster or podium presentations at local, regional, national and international levels.

- **Teaching experience**

  Most doctors would have conducted some form of informal teaching at some point. Hence, getting involved in formal teaching (such as organising FY1 lunchtime teachings, medical student prescribing tutorials or department journal clubs) will make your CV stand out.

- **Leadership and teamwork**

  In this section, list your positions of responsibility and provide examples of your organisational and team working skills in achieving a desired outcome (may be medical or non-medical).

- **Other competency questions**

  Consider answering questions by first providing a *scenario*, then explaining the *action* taken (and demonstrating the tested attribute), and finally describing the *outcome* of your action.

Other questions may be designed to assess your suitability for a surgical specialty, such as evidence of hand-eye coordination (e.g. the ability to play racquet games or musical instruments to a reasonable standard). Keeping a logbook of interesting communication situations with patients and colleagues will come in handy when asked to demonstrate problem-solving and leadership skills. Finally, get involved in organising rotas and seminars to show your management skills.

Shortlisting

Your application form will only be assessed if it is correctly completed and submitted. If you fulfil all the eligibility requirements, your application will then be scored against the national person specification. If you are among the highest scoring applicants, you will be invited to attend the interview. Generally, there will be more applicants shortlisted than there are OST1 posts.

Only shortlisted applicants will be contacted. You will not be contacted if you have not made the shortlist. If you have not heard by the interview date, you can assume that your application has not been successful and that you have not been shortlisted.

You can request for feedback regarding your application if you have not been shortlisted. You can do so via email or post, and the request must include your full name, GMC number, and the OST level that you applied for. Those who request for feedback will receive a copy of the following:

- Rank and / or score
- Total number of applicants
- Rank and / or score required to be shortlisted for interview

You can go through a complaints procedure if you have any concerns about your application or if you feel that your application has been wrongly or unfairly scored.

For more about feedback and the complaints procedure, please visit:
http://www.mmc.nhs.uk/specialty_training/specialty_training_2012/feedback_complaints/requesting_feedback.aspx
http://www.mmc.nhs.uk/specialty_training_2013/specialty_training_2013/feedback_complaints/a_fair_process.aspx

You do not have much time between shortlisting and attending interviews, so be prepared early. Do not take your foot off the pedal after shortlisting, and if anything, you should work even harder to hone your interview skills.

Interviews

The purpose of the interview is to assess your suitability for an OST post and to make sure that you meet the required person specification criteria. Interviews usually take at least 60 minutes. The interview panel members will score each candidate based on interview performance and the highest scoring candidates will be offered OST posts.

All being well, you will have impressed the interview panel sufficiently for them to offer you that coveted OST1 post at your preferred Postgraduate Deanery. If you were unsuccessful, you can request for feedback on your interview and information regarding your interview score.

For advice on interview preparation, performance and feedback, please refer to Chapter 4.

Offers

OST posts are matched as best as possible to candidates' preferences. This means that offers are made to candidates who ranked highest in the interview who also ranked a particular Postgraduate Deanery the highest. If you are successful in your interview, you will be contacted with news of an offer in February or March. You may receive an offer after March if higher-scoring candidates reject their offer.

Notification of offers for OST posts are sent to your email address via the **UK Offers System** (https://www.ukoffers.org.uk/Login.aspx). When you apply for an OST post, you will be requested to log in to the UK Offers System, set up a password and check your contact email details. This system allows you to rank your preferred Postgraduate Deaneries online. The higher your interview score, the higher your chances of being offered an OST1 position at your preferred Postgraduate Deanery.

When you receive an offer, you have 48 hours (including weekends and bank holidays) to decide if you want to accept, reject or hold the offer. If you do not respond within 48 hours, the offer to you will be withdrawn and subsequently offered to another applicant.

Sometimes, there may be personal or family issues that require further consideration before you can accept an offer. Check with the Postgraduate Deanery how long you are allowed to hold an offer for – if you do not accept the offer within the specified time limit, you will be considered to have rejected the offer. You can only hold 1 offer at a time.

Similarly, you cannot accept more than 1 offer at the same time. Once you have accepted an offer, you cannot accept other offers and you will need to withdraw from all your other applications. However, there is an exception to this rule: you will still be eligible to apply for an ACF post even if you have already accepted an OST1 post.

The Next Step

Your future employer will run pre-employment checks on you before you receive an offer of employment. The aim of pre-employment checks is to ensure that you are fit and safe to work with patients. These include immigration status checks, English language proficiency, verification of references, update on GMC licence to practise, occupational health clearance, and Criminal Records Bureau disclosures.

Your offer of employment will include information such as:

- Contact details for further information
- Your place of work, start date, and duration of the post
- Working hours, pattern of work and duty hours, and out of hours rota
- Basic pay as described by national salary scales
- Any specific pay supplement, London weighting or recruitment incentive
- Pension arrangements and notice period
- Annual leave entitlement, statutory days and study leave arrangements
- Sick pay arrangements with reference to national terms and conditions
- Requirements of pre-employment procedures and checks
- Professional registration requirements
- Local policies on health and safety
- Proposed salary deductions, such as mess fees
- Educational Supervisor and Clinical Tutor
- Accommodation details
- Induction arrangements for newly starting doctors

Your offer of employment is separate from your OST programme training agreement with the Postgraduate Deanery. Over the course of your OST programme, you may change employers (and work in different hospitals) a few times. Each new employer will likely conduct pre-employment checks on you before you start work with them. If you are unable to commence work on the designated start date, inform your future employer well in advance so they can make alternative arrangements.

Chapter 4

The Interview Process

Shi Zhuan Tan

Ken Lee Lai

Brian Ang

The Interview Process

Congratulations! You have been selected for the all-important interview. All your hard work thus far has paid off, and you now have the chance to present to the interview panel what you can do and why you deserve the OST post. At this critical point, it cannot be stressed enough the importance of meticulous preparation for the interview. Candidates tend to spend a lot of time and effort building up their CVs and filling in the application forms, but the time and effort dedicated to interview preparation is woefully inadequate.

Remember that the interview carries a lot of weight. So if anything, you should spend as much time on interview preparation as you would on the applications process. Once shortlisted for the interview, you are considered on par with the other selected candidates. At this stage, it doesn't matter how many publications you have – you still need to perform on that day! You need to impress and show that you are the best candidate for the job.

To ensure your greatest chance of performing well, it is *crucial* to know the format of the interview. It allows you to prepare accordingly, and avoids any potential unwelcome surprises. The interview may involve a single panel interview and / or multiple stations.

Example stations include:
- **Clinical scenario stations**
  - Management of a clinical condition
  - Asking for advice from a consultant over the telephone
  - Obtaining informed consent
  - Preparing a discharge summary
- **Clinical skills stations**
  - Suturing
  - Tests of hand-eye coordination
- **Research, audit and critical appraisal station**
- **Portfolio and CV station**

Interview Format

At the time of print (2013), recruitment for OST is conducted by the Severn Deanery on behalf of the Royal College of Ophthalmologists. Interviews are held in Bristol over a period of 3 days.

The interview format for the year 2013 includes 4 stations which are as follows:

- **Critical appraisal station** (25 minutes)
- **Structured interview – communication station** (12 minutes)
- **Structured interview – clinical scenario station** (12 minutes)
- **Structured interview – portfolio review station** (12 minutes)

Past questions about the OST1 national recruitment interview can be found at: http://www.eyedocs.co.uk/ophthalmology-interview-feedback-st/607-st1-national-recruitment-interview-

For other example interview questions, please refer to the Appendices section of the book.

Do be aware that the interview format and questions may change from year to year, so make sure you clarify with the Postgraduate Deanery once you have been shortlisted for interview.

Pre-Interview Preparation

Your interview preparations should be similar whether the interview is for a clinical or academic training post. Bear in mind that the purpose of the interview is to assess your interest and suitability in a career in ophthalmology. The interview panel will want to find out if you meet (or exceed) the person specifications for OST1, and then select only the best candidates for the posts.

To impress your interviewers and to do well in your interview, you need to be able to deliver answers in a polished and systematic manner. It is therefore vital that your preparations should include interview practice as well as efforts to demonstrate that you are indeed keen and ideally suited to take up an OST1 post.

- **Interview skills courses**

  Interview skills courses are great at providing interview practice as well as up-to-date information regarding possible interview topics. Most applicants attending interview courses have found them to be very beneficial, particularly the experience of going through the mock interviews. However, do be aware that most courses are generic in nature and may not specifically be tailored for ophthalmology.

  Some of the more popular interview skills courses include:

  - *Ophthalmology ST Interview Skills Course*
    http://ophthcourse.webs.com

  - *Hammersmith Interview Skills Course*
    http://www.medicalcommunicationskills.com/specialty_interviews.html

  - *Interview Skills for Junior Doctors*
    http://bma.org.uk/events/2013/tag/interview-skills-for-junior-doctors

  - *Oxford Medical ST Interview Course*
    http://www.medicalinterviewsuk.co.uk/st-interview-course.html

- **Practice, practice, practice**

  Unfortunately, self-promotion and attendance at interview skills courses alone are insufficient to land you the OST post that you desire. The acid test occurs during the interview, and you need to be well-drilled in facing the various components of different interview formats. As it is virtually impossible to predict what will be asked during the interview, it is therefore important to prepare answers to standard questions that are likely to be asked and have been asked before. Bear in mind that it is the framework and approach to answering questions that will be of help to you. Have a logical sequence in mind when tackling questions.

  In this respect, the importance of practice and yet more practice cannot be overemphasised. Focus your efforts in the following areas:

  - *Interview answer delivery*

    There is no better preparation than to rehearse your answers repeatedly until you have an auto-cue running in your head. Your answers should flow easily and naturally. Prepare cue cards containing key points for each question, and then practise expanding on those key words. Verbalise your answers in front of a mirror. Focus on your articulation and intonation. Practising in front of friends or colleagues allows you to obtain feedback on your performance. Ask them to highlight any mannerisms or body language that does not project a sense of professionalism and confidence. This is definitely the time to get rid of any distracting hand gestures and irritating verbal interjections. Having your interview practice sessions videotaped is an excellent (albeit potentially embarrassing) way of gaining insight into how you are actually seen and heard by the interviewers. When you feel more confident, try to arrange a mock interview with your mentors, current senior colleagues or local consultant ophthalmologists. This exercise is invaluable as it will prepare you mentally for what it would be like on the interview day itself.

- *Suturing and surgical instrument handling*

    The basic skills involved in using the operating microscope and microsurgical instruments are covered in the **Basic Microsurgical Skills Course** organised by the Royal College of Ophthalmologists. If you are unable to attend the course, try to borrow the course manual from someone who has. Attending ophthalmology theatre sessions allows you to see how the instruments are handled and used. However, just merely looking is not enough, so make sure you that you do practice handling surgical instruments and tying simple interrupted sutures on sponges or tomatoes. Your mentors or local consultant ophthalmologists should be able to advise you on your surgical technique and on how to procure instruments.

- *Critical appraisal*

    You will need to know how to critically appraise a scientific article. In the critical appraisal station, you will usually be given 20 to 40 minutes to read a manuscript, and then 5 to 10 minutes to present your appraisal. The interviewers will then ask you a series of questions regarding that paper, including research methodology. Ask your mentors or senior colleagues to select several papers for you to critically appraise, and then present your appraisal to them. You will also get excellent practice by actively participating in journal club sessions. Appraise all articles in the same systematic way so that it becomes second nature.

Start practising as soon as the application is submitted – there will usually be **no more than 2 to 4 weeks** from shortlisting to the day the interview is conducted. Get as much constructive criticism and feedback as possible. This is the time to put ego aside and take on board all relevant advice and suggestions. Do not be shy to ask for help and advice from those who have gone through the process before – you'll be amazed at how much you will learn.

- **Answer preparation**

  In the past, interviews were set up to gauge your commitment to ophthalmology and to evaluate your personality as a work colleague. Interviews have now evolved to include assessment of your aptitude, clinical knowledge, surgical skills, and reasoning and appraisal ability. It is thus crucial that you prepare yourself well in these areas:

  - *Clinical knowledge*

    Familiarise yourself with the management and counselling of common eye problems (cataract; glaucoma; etc) and ocular emergencies (acute primary angle closure; chemical injury, etc).

  - *Clinical governance*

    http://www.bmj.com/content/317/7150/61

    You will need to know the definitions of the various components that comprise clinical governance (please see the Glossary section in the Appendices chapter). Clinical governance topics are usually well covered at most interview skills courses.

  - *Suture material and surgical instruments*

    http://www.mrcophth.com/eyesurgery.htm

    Make sure you have basic knowledge of the various suture and needle types, as well as their indications and advantages. These are covered in the **Basic Microsurgical Skills Course** organised by the Royal College of Ophthalmologists. Knowledge of cataract surgery principles would also be advantageous.

  - *Critical appraisal*

    http://www.bmj.com/about-bmj/resources-readers/publications/statistics-square-one

    To appraise critically, you must have an understanding of basic research and statistical principles. If you have time, read up on study design, sample size calculation, types of bias, ethics considerations, *P*-values, and 95% confidence intervals.

You may also find the following pre-interview preparation steps useful, although they are more applicable for interviews conducted by individual Postgraduate Deaneries rather than nationally-conducted interviews.

- **Information gathering**

  Find out about the rotation and the various departments that you would be expected to spend part of your training in. Information is usually available from the application forms and the Postgraduate Deanery websites. Often, a different perspective can be gained from speaking to the local ophthalmology trainees. This can be arranged via the department secretary or simply by calling the on-call ophthalmology trainee (during reasonable hours). Find out about the post, working environment, quality of training and interview format.

- **Hospital visits**

  If possible, go the extra mile and visit the different eye units prior to the interview. This shows interest on your part, and also provides an idea of what it would be like working in those units. Inform the secretary of the department that you would like to visit and make a mutually suitable appointment. Often, postgraduate teaching sessions are good times to visit because most of the consultants (including the ones who may be involved in the interview) are likely to be present. However, visits to all units may not be feasible so you may have to prioritise your approach and perhaps visit the main teaching centre and one other larger regional department.

- **Contact with senior managers in ophthalmology**

  This is not something that many shortlisted candidates think of doing. By speaking to the senior managers, you may gain an insight into any forthcoming developments in the local eye department or any new approaches to local eye care delivery. Having obtained up-to-date information about local eye services, you will sound very impressive when discussing how that particular department might evolve in the future and how you may be able to contribute to it.

- **Contact with consultant ophthalmologists**

  You should be able to find the names of the relevant consultant ophthalmologists and the appropriate contact details from the application forms. You may also ring up the personnel department or the department secretaries to ask if they can suggest any other consultants who will be or have been involved with the interview process. Generally most departments will provide a list of potential interviewers. Your aim is to ease yourself into the awareness of these consultants without being intrusive. However, please do not force the issue as they will also be very busy with their own work.

  You can do this in several ways, including:
  - *Hospital visits*

    It is unlikely that you will have the opportunity to arrange a formal visit specifically to speak to the consultant ophthalmologists involved in the interview. However, when you do make your informal hospital visit, you may bump into them during the teaching session or somewhere in the department. If you do meet them, be mindful that their time is limited. So keep things concise and to the point. Impress upon them your keen interest in the job and thank them for taking the time to speak to you.

  - *Email*

    If you are not able to visit any units, convey your interest in the job via email once you have permission (via their secretaries) to contact them. Attach your CV and make sure you include a picture profile so that they can put a face to your name.

  - *Consultant to consultant*

    Do not underestimate the power of a glowing endorsement from your mentor or current consultant to his or her friend or previous colleague working in the Postgraduate Deanery that you've been shortlisted for. It is natural tendency for people to be more likely to accept recommendations from someone they know personally.

Before the Interview Day

To make the whole process as stress-free as possible, there are several things that you need to take care of prior to the interview:

- **Timing**. This may sound obvious, but make sure you confirm the date and time of your interview. Once confirmed, give as much notice as you can to your workplace so that your clinical and administrative colleagues know of your impending absence. Make the necessary arrangements and swaps for your on-calls and clinic sessions. Interviews often run late, so try not to schedule a shift or on-call duty immediately after the scheduled interview end time.

- **Location**. This is again obvious, but extremely important. Make sure you enquire and confirm the exact location and venue of your interview. Note down a contact telephone number for the venue, just in case you need directions on the day. Nothing is worse than turning up late for the interview feeling flustered, disorientated and apologetic, just because you ended up going to the wrong venue. Look up the address on Google maps and plan your transport options in advance, taking into account the traffic and interview time. Depending on how far you have to travel, you may have to book coach, rail, ferry or air tickets, as well as overnight accommodation. If possible, make a trial visit to the venue so you know exactly how to get there, where to park and how long the journey takes.

- **Essential documents**. Finally, double check that you have in your possession all documents that may be required for the interview. Collate all the documentation (passport, logbook, certificates, portfolio, etc) in an interview folder. You don't really want to be panicking the night before the interview desperately searching for the certificates that you were convinced were located in some drawer somewhere. You must be prepared to provide evidence for any and every statement made on your CV and application form.

The Interview Day

Well, the big day has now arrived! All the hard work has been done – you have gotten yourself shortlisted for interview, and you have practised and practised your interview answers and technique. This is the day that you put all that you have learnt into practice. You will most likely be nervous, but don't worry; if you have put in the effort, you are likely to perform well. There are 3 parts to consider on the actual interview day:

- **Getting ready before the interview**
  - *Dress smart.* How you look is often the first impression the interviewers have of you. There is no harm in putting in the extra effort to look more professional. Make sure you wear a smart suit, a finely pressed light-coloured or white shirt, and polished dark shoes. Brush your teeth and comb your hair before leaving home. When you look good, you feel good. Gentlemen, please refrain from wearing a cartoon or flamboyant necktie, even if the necktie is your lucky charm. Ladies, please avoid complicated colours and risqué styles, however much you feel that it is your right to express yourself.

  - *Essential documents.* Bring all your essential documents and copies of those documents. These include your passport, visa grant letter, English qualifications, GMC certificate, trainers' reports, logbook, certificates, audits, publications, written workplace assessments, and portfolio. If you are unsure, just bring the document along anyway for peace of mind.

  - *Arrive early.* Arrive at least 30 minutes before your interview start time. Take into account traffic, parking, and any potential delays on your way to the interview venue. One of the worst things you can do is to arrive late and then be flustered during the interview. Arriving early allows you to go to the washroom and to freshen up. To help calm your nerves, have a walk around, chat with other candidates, or pick a quiet spot to meditate and relax.

- **Performing during the interview**
  - *Smile!* The moment you step into the room is the moment that your interviewers form an immediate impression of you. When you are asked to enter, tidy up smartly and walk confidently into the room. Greet your interviewers with a big warm smile and small courteous nods. Do maintain a straight and natural posture. Whatever you do, please do not carry yourself in a lazy and disinterested manner or keep your gaze fixed on the ground. Respond to each introduction with a smile and an assured "Hello". A smiling face is a lot easier to like than a sullen one. Although you will be anxious, try to *appear pleasant all the time*. The interviewers will be using this opportunity to determine if you are a colleague that they will be comfortable working with.

  - *Handshake.* Try not to be overly enthusiastic and aggressive in your approach. Give a firm and positive handshake when initiated by the interview panel. Remember that the aim of the handshake is to transmit confidence and not to crush the hands of your interviewers.

  - *Sitting posture.* Sit on the chair with an upright but relaxed posture. A slight forward lean demonstrates a studied interest over a point of discussion. A slight backward lean displays a sense of professional calmness. Whatever your sitting preference, *do not slouch* in your chair. At this stage, you will also likely be conscious as to what to do with your hands. The best suggestion is to put your hands on your lap with your fingers interlaced. This will reduce any tendency to keep flicking your hair or adjusting your spectacles. Avoid gripping the arm rests or your lap so tightly to the extent that your knuckles become white. Do not stretch your legs out too much, and watch that you do not shake your legs or shift them too often.

- *Answer delivery.* **Speak clearly and confidently.** Do not mumble your answers because no one will be impressed, not least the interviewers. By all means, take a brief moment to think of your answers to avoid saying something that you should not have. It is alright to have pauses in between answering, especially when you are faced with a challenging question. Do not be afraid to ask the interviewers to clarify or rephrase the question if you're unclear. Paraphrasing the question is an excellent way to confirm your understanding of what is being asked. It also buys you a few extra precious seconds to gather your thoughts and provide an answer. Whatever you do, please do not argue with the interview panel, even if you are 100% certain that the interviewers are wrong!

- *Hand gestures.* It is perfectly acceptable to use small and simple hand gestures to emphasise certain points and reinforce your delivery. They can also help to regulate and pace your answers. However, please do not be too theatrical in your gesticulations as they will only serve to distract yourself and the interview panel.

- *Articulation.* Maintain a good energy and volume throughout your sentences. Watch that your voice does not trail off towards the end of an answer, and be careful not to answer the questions in the manner of a speeding train. These are natural tendencies when nervousness and anxiety sets in. When you have finished your answer, end on a confident note instead of dragging it out.

- *Eye contact and head nodding.* Demonstrate that you are interested and enthusiastic during the interview. Always **maintain good eye contact** with every member of the interview panel, and not just the person asking you the question. This way, you actively draw in the entire panel while you speak. Nod appropriately to show that you are listening attentively to what is being said and asked.

- **Bowing out after the interview**

  - *Questions.* At the end of the interview, the panel will often provide an indication of when the results will be announced. You will then subsequently be asked if you have any questions for the interview panel. If you feel that you have done your best and that there is nothing else you need to clarify, then a simple "No, thank you" will suffice. On the other hand, if you feel that there has been a glaring omission from your interview, then this is your opportunity to highlight it to the interviewers. You may deliver a small statement to reaffirm your commitment towards the post. While it may not change the outcome of the interview, a positive end statement from you may be appreciated more than you think. A reasonable question to ask is how you can obtain feedback from the interview panel. Please do not waste the interviewers' time by asking questions that are better answered by someone else. These include questions on claiming back your interview travel expenses or paternity leave allowance for that particular Postgraduate Deanery.

  - *Thank the interviewers.* Regardless of how you feel you have been treated during the interview, it is only polite that you thank the interviewers as you leave the room. Do so courteously. After all, the panel will have faced or will be facing a long hard day interviewing candidates. Hopefully, you would have made their task tougher by performing impressively during the interview.

  - *Contact details.* Leave your contact number and email address with the administrator present at the interview; this allows the Postgraduate Deanery to contact you easily at short notice.

  - *Receipts.* Keep your receipts as you may be able to claim back the expenses incurred while travelling to attend the interview. Not all costs will be reimbursed, so do check with the interview administrator.

What Interviewers Look For

While it may seem a bit presumptuous, it is worthwhile putting yourself in the shoes of the interviewers. Just imagine that you are one of the consultant ophthalmologists in the interview panel: What would *you* be trying to find out from a candidate during the interview that you do not already know from the application form or CV? What type of trainee would you like to spend your time working with and train?

In general, there are 3 important characteristics that interviewers look for:

- **Confidence**. Interviewers like candidates who are confident. Having confidence in yourself will instil confidence in the interviewers. Consultants love trainees who are confident within the limits of their own clinical and surgical skills. However, please do not confuse this with arrogance – arrogance is a turn-off and is an absolute no-no. This is because consultants also want to be confident that whoever they appoint will seek senior advice when appropriate. Nobody wants brash loose cannons as trainees in their department.

- **Ability to work well in a team**. Like it or not, as a trainee, you will need to work with other ophthalmology colleagues (junior and senior), colleagues in other medical and surgical specialties, as well as allied healthcare professionals. This can sometimes be difficult due to differences in personality, especially in high pressure, stressful situations. Interviewers will want to know if you are professional enough to be able to put aside personal differences for the benefit of the patient and the team.

- **Enthusiasm**. Enthusiasm can be very infectious. Consultants love to mentor and teach enthusiastic trainees who go the extra mile for their own training and in the course of providing care for patients. Try to convey your enthusiasm to the interviewers, and better still, provide some examples of how your enthusiasm has led to a change where you have worked previously.

Interview Feedback

Successful or not, it is a good idea to ask for feedback regarding your performance during the interview. This can be done by sending a written or email request to the relevant Postgraduate Deanery.

If you request for interview feedback, you will receive a copy of the following information within 40 days:

- Rank and / or score
- Total number of candidates interviewed
- Rank and / or score required to receive an offer

You can also request for copies of your interview score sheets. These will be handled by the Postgraduate Deanery in line with the Data Protection Act.

Chapter 5

The Unsuccessful Applicant

Brian Ang

The Unsuccessful Applicant

Don't be too downcast or down-hearted. This is the nature of competitive specialties, and there will always be both successful and unsuccessful applicants. Keep your chin up, and keep persevering. Think of it as an opportunity to do something that hopefully you will enjoy and will also bolster your CV.

In the past, SHO posts in specialties such as Neurology, Neurosurgery and Accident & Emergency were routes to getting into ophthalmology. It bought time, skills and experience while waiting to land that elusive ophthalmology registrar training post. Others have taken on medical posts or pursued academic higher degrees, spending 2 to 4 years doing research. The more adventurous go off the beaten track and spend time being involved with eye-related charities in developing countries.

Whatever you choose to do, you should use this time wisely. Fill up any gaps in your CV and portfolio, and correct any weaknesses that were highlighted to you in your previous application. You will also need to be able to justify how you spent your year and how it has been beneficial for you. People you can obtain practical careers advice from, include:

- Your mentor(s)
- Your Educational Supervisor
- The Clinical Tutor in your local hospital
- The Director of Medical Education in your local hospital
- The British Medical Association (BMA) Careers Guidance Service
  http://bma.org.uk/developing-your-career

In this chapter, we discuss some of the different options available to you while waiting for the next recruitment window for OST applications, including:

- Non-OST posts
- Medical posts
- Higher academic degrees
- Pursue training abroad

Non-OST Posts

These temporary posts are useful as they help you gain skills and experience while awaiting the next round of OST applications. Such posts may be advertised in the classifieds section of the British Medical Journal.

- **Non-OST ophthalmology posts**

  Although the number of ophthalmology training posts has decreased, the overall workload has in fact increased. To cope with the increased demand, various long-term and short-term non-training posts have been created; these generally involve ward work, preoperative assessment and eye casualty. As they are not OST posts, you may not have any opportunities for surgery. Try not to be in such posts for more than 18 months as it may reduce your chances of entering into an OST programme (too experienced for OST1; or perceived as not being able to make the grade out of "dead end" non-training posts). There are 3 types of such posts:

  - *Locum Appointment for Training (LAT)*

    These short-term posts can be counted towards the CCT. Appointments to LAT posts can only be made by a formally-defined appointments panel.

  - *Locum Appointment for Service (LAS)*

    These short-term posts do not count towards the CCT. Appointments are less formal and are made by the local hospital.

  - *Trust Grade*

    These long-term posts do not count towards the CCT. Appointments are less formal and are made by the local hospital.

- **Posts in related specialties**

  Locum posts in related specialties (*Accident & Emergency, Neurology, Neurosurgery, Endocrinology, Rheumatology*) are popular for those wanting experience that would benefit their future OST application. However, these posts are in short supply and are competitive in their own right.

Medical Posts

The 2 main benefits of medical posts are the MRCP qualification and the option to enter into a career in Medical Ophthalmology.

- **MRCP (Membership of the Royal College of Physicians)**
  http://www.mrcpuk.org/Pages/Home.aspx
  The Part 1 written examination can be taken at any time after graduation from medical school. The Part 2 consists of a written component and a clinical component (PACES), both of which must be taken within 7 years of passing the Part 1. It is recommended that candidates should have some medical experience first, such as that gained from *Core Medical Training*, before attempting PACES. This would involve entering *Core Medical Training* initially, either on a locum or permanent basis, and then after successful completion of the MRCP, to reapply for the next OST programme.

- **Medical Ophthalmology**
  http://www.jrcptb.org.uk/trainingandcert/ST3-SpR/Pages/Medical-Ophthalmology.aspx
  http://careers.bmj.com/careers/advice/view-article.html?id=2902
  For trainees who choose to complete *Core Medical Training*, there is the option of pursuing a career in Medical Ophthalmology. Medical Ophthalmology is a relatively new specialty that deals with the medical management of ocular problems secondary to systemic disease (e.g. diabetic retinopathy, thyroid eye disease, giant cell arteritis, etc), and therefore does not include any surgical training. The MRCP is mandatory for training in Medical Ophthalmology. The training in this field is overseen by a joint committee comprising physicians and ophthalmologists under the Joint Royal Colleges of Physicians Training Board, and NOT by the Royal College of Ophthalmologists. Those who choose this option usually do not return to surgical training in OST.

Higher Academic Degrees

Higher academic degrees, either taught or by research, are excellent ways of enhancing your CV. Traditionally, most would enter science and research based higher degrees (MSc / MD / PhD), although there are now some who prefer a management-related qualification (MBA). However, these degrees will incur a very significant time and cost commitment.

- **MSc (Master of Science)**

  MSc degrees can be done either full time or part time, over 1 to 5 years. An MSc degree may be clinical, laboratory or informatics based, and will provide a solid grounding for designing and conducting research in the future. For those even more academically inclined, the MSc will be an excellent platform to subsequently pursue a PhD degree.

  Listed below are some MSc programmes related to ophthalmology:

  - *MSc Biology of Vision (Institute of Ophthalmology, London)*
    http://www.ucl.ac.uk/ioo-courses/msc-bov

  - *MSc Clinical Ophthalmology (Institute of Ophthalmology, London)*
    http://www.ucl.ac.uk/ioo-courses/msc-co

  - *MSc Ophthalmology Retina or Cataract & Refractive Surgery (Institute of Ophthalmology, London)*
    http://www.ucl.ac.uk/ioo-courses/msc-o-r

  - *MSc Clinical Ophthalmology and Vision Research (Glasgow Caledonian University, Glasgow)*
    http://www.gcu.ac.uk/study/postgraduate/courses/clinical-ophthalmology-and-vision-research-generic-9524.php?loc=uk

  - *MSc Investigative Ophthalmology and Vision Sciences (University of Manchester)*
    http://www.mhs.manchester.ac.uk/postgraduate/programmes/taughtmasters/ophthalmology

- **MD (Doctor of Medicine) / PhD (Doctor of Philosophy)**

  Consider this option if you have a strong interest in academia, especially if you intend to combine clinical work with research in your practice. Academic ophthalmologists are clinician-scientists, and most will have completed an MD or PhD degree at some point in their careers. MDs can take 2 to 3 years while PhDs can take 3 to 4 years. These will require a substantial investment in terms of time and money. For this reason, it is important that you pick a research topic that you are genuinely interested in and a supervisor that you can get along with.

  Listed below is a selection of programmes that you may consider:

  - *MD / PhD Eye & Vision Sciences (University of Liverpool)*
    http://www.liv.ac.uk/ageing-and-chronic-disease/postgraduate/phd-mphil-study/eye-and-vision-sciences-mphil-phd-md/overview

  - *PhD Ophthalmology (University of Manchester)*
    http://www.manchester.ac.uk/postgraduate/researchdegrees/researchdegrees/bysubject/03127/ophthalmology-phd

  - *PhD Clinical Ophthalmology (Institute of Ophthalmology, London)*
    http://www.ucl.ac.uk/ioo/jobs/clinphdprog.htm

  - *PhD Visual Neuroscience & Molecular Biology (Cardiff University)*
    http://courses.cardiff.ac.uk/postgraduate/course/detail/p318.html.html

  It is not necessary for the MD / PhD research topics to be directly related to ophthalmology. Other relevant research areas include:
  - *Healthcare Management*
  - *Epidemiology & Public Health*
  - *Medical Education*
  - *Health Informatics*
  - *Clinical Neuroscience*

- **MBA (Master of Business Administration)**

  An MBA gives you a different dimension as it focuses on delivering results through effective management. It is ideal if you would like to focus on management in the clinical setting later on in your career. It may also be used as a stepping stone towards a hospital management career or work in the private sector (private healthcare organisations, medical device and pharmaceutical companies, etc). Many MBA programmes are available.

  Programmes relevant to healthcare management include:
  - *MBA Healthcare Management (University of East London)*
    http://www.uel.ac.uk/study/courses/healthcareman.htm
  - *MBA Healthcare Management (Brunel University, London)*
    http://www.brunel.ac.uk/bbs/mba/mba-specialisations/healthcare-management
  - *MBA Healthcare (University of Bedfordshire)*
    https://www.beds.ac.uk/howtoapply/courses/postgraduate/business-administration-healthcare
  - *Health Executive MBA (Keele University)*
    http://www.keele.ac.uk/pgtcourses/healthexecutivemba
  - *MBA in Hospital Management (Anglia Ruskin University)*
    http://www.anglia.ac.uk/ruskin/en/home/faculties/fhsce/postgraduate/mba_hospital_admin.html
  - *MBA in Leadership and Management in Healthcare (Canterbury Christ Church University)*
    http://www.canterbury.ac.uk/courses/prospectus/postgraduate/courses/mba_health.asp
  - *Executive MBA Healthcare (University of Nottingham)*
    http://www.asgbi.org.uk/en/postgraduate_qualifications/executive_mba_healthcare__nottingham_university.cfm

Pursue Training Abroad

Finally, if all else fails, you can always consider the option of going abroad to gain entry into an overseas ophthalmology training programme. Although attractive, there are 2 main issues to consider before uprooting yourself.

Firstly, the UK medical degree may not be recognised and you may need to sit for the medical examinations of the country you wish to practice in. For instance, to pursue ophthalmology training in the United States (US), you must first pass the **United States Medical Licensing Examination** comprising 3 exam parts (USMLE; http://www.usmle.org), before you can practise as a medical doctor. For more about US residency programmes, visit: http://www.facs.org/residencysearch/specialties/ophthal.html

Secondly, as in the UK, competition for these posts is also very stiff and usually only residents and citizens are allowed to apply. This means that you'll need to have spent a few years in the country to gain resident status first before being eligible to enter into training posts. For example, to enter into a training programme under the **Royal Australian & New Zealand College of Ophthalmologists**, you need to fulfil the following requirements (http://www.ranzco.edu/index.php/about/training/vocational-training/how-to-apply):

- Australian or New Zealand citizen or permanent resident
- Full registration to practise medicine in Australia or New Zealand
- Minimum 2 years of non-ophthalmology postgraduate experience
- Postgraduate qualification (not essential, but a definite advantage)
    - *Graduate Diploma in Ophthalmic Science (University of Sydney)*
      http://sydney.edu.au/courses/Graduate-Diploma-in-Ophthalmic-Science
    - *Master of Ophthalmology (University of Otago)*
      http://www.otago.ac.nz/courses/qualifications/mophth.html
    - *Masters of Ophthalmology (University of Adelaide)*
      http://health.adelaide.edu.au/ophthalmology/post_graduate/masters.html

The decision to go abroad to pursue your dream of becoming an ophthalmologist is not an easy one to make, although the experience is often very worthwhile. But please be aware that this will involve plenty of administrative and bureaucratic paperwork. You will definitely need to set aside some *money (at least £2,000)* and *time (at least 6 months)*. To work in Australia or New Zealand (NZ), these are the administrative issues that a junior doctor typically has to go through:

- **Securing a post**

  You are extremely unlikely to waltz right into an ophthalmology registrar training programme. More likely, you will be working in a non-training ophthalmology post in a more rural location or in a related specialty. There are many medical recruitment agencies that will help you search for ophthalmology posts in Australia and NZ.

- **Australian Medical Council / Medical Council of New Zealand**
  http://www.amc.org.au; http://www.mcnz.org.nz

  To register with the medical councils, you will need to send in the completed relevant application forms and documentary evidence of the following (all photocopies must be certified by a notary public):

  - Job offer letter and job description
  - Letters of appointments from previous jobs
  - Medical degree and other qualifications
  - Proficiency in written and spoken English

    (International English Language Testing System – IELTS): http://www.ielts.org/default.aspx

  - GMC and other medical council registration
  - GMC Certificate of Good Standing:
    http://www.gmc-uk.org/cgs_online
  - Evidence of medical indemnity: http://www.medicalprotection.org

  - Passport sized photographs, certified behind by a notary public
  - Passport details page, including the signature page
  - Driving licence as another form of photo identification

- **Visa / Work permit application**

  http://www.immi.gov.au; http://www.immigration.govt.nz

  To enter the country to work, you will need to have the relevant visa or work permit. If you are unsure of which application forms to submit, please contact the relevant immigration authorities. You will need to send in the completed application forms as well as evidence of the following (all photocopies must be certified by a notary public):

  - Job offer letter and job description
  - Medical degree and other qualifications
  - Australian Medical Council / Medical Council of NZ registration
  - Proficiency in written and spoken English **(International English Language Testing System – IELTS)**:

    http://www.ielts.org/default.aspx

  - Full medical check-up by approved general practitioners
  - Blood tests (including HIV, hepatitis B and C, syphilis) by approved labs
  - Chest X-ray by approved radiology centres
  - **UK Police Certificate**:

    http://www.acro.police.uk/police_certificates.aspx

  - **Certificate of Good Conduct** or **Record of Criminal Convictions** from your home country
  - Passport sized photographs, certified behind by a notary public
  - Passport details page, including the signature page
  - Driving licence
  - Bank statements and evidence of funds
  - Proof of address (utility bills, credit card statements, etc)

  There are stringent criteria for passport photograph acceptance, as well as for how photocopies of documents and passport photographs are certified. It will be extremely frustrating if your applications are rejected purely on the grounds of not adhering to these guidelines. Send completed applications by registered mail for peace of mind.

Appendices

Example CV

Personal & Contact Details

- Name: Amy Loid
- Current Position: Foundation Year 2 Doctor
- Date of Birth: 8th August 1988
- GMC registration:
- Professional address: Royal Infirmary of Edinburgh
- Telephone number:
- Email address: amy.loid@nhs.net

Education & Professional Qualifications

- FRCOphth Part 1, Royal College of Ophthalmologists, (Date)
- ICO Basic Science Exam, International Council of Ophthalmology, (Date)
- MBChB, University of Edinburgh Medical School, (Date)

Achievements & Awards

- 10th Place Duke Elder Undergraduate Ophthalmology Prize, (Date)
- Wellcome Trust Student Elective Prize, (Date)
- Royal College of Ophthalmologists Trevor-Roper Travel Award, (Date)
- University of Edinburgh Elective Bursary Award, (Date)
- University of Edinburgh MacKenzie Bursary in Anatomy, (Date)

Elective & Special Study Module

- Elective: Wills Eye Institute, Philadephia. Supervisor: (Name)
  Describe your experience and what you learnt

- SSM: Moorfields Eye Hospital, London. Supervisor: (Name)
  Project title:
  Describe your experience and what you learnt

Employment History

- Current position: (Hospital), (Date)
- Previous positions: (Hospital), (Date)

Portfolio

- Foundation Year learning outcomes: All achieved
- OST1 learning outcomes: 3 achieved (PS11, PS22, SS2)

Ophthalmology Experience

- Taster week in ophthalmology at St. Paul's Eye Unit, Liverpool
- During my free time, I attended ophthalmology clinics and theatre as an observer at the Princess Alexandra Eye Pavilion, Edinburgh
- Competent in slit lamp examination and Goldmann tonometry

Courses

- Royal College of Ophthalmologists Basic Microsurgical Skills Course, (Date)
- Edinburgh FOCUS – Foundation Course in Ophthalmology, (Date)
- Communication Skills Course, (Date)
- Statistics for Clinicians Course, (Date)
- Advanced Life Support, (Date)

Publications

- Loid A. Title of paper. Eye News 2010
- Loid A. Title of paper. In press: Eye 2010

Presentations

- Scottish Ophthalmological Club Meeting: Podium presentation, (Date) Title of presentation. Loid A.

- Royal College of Ophthalmologists Annual Congress: Poster, (Date) Title of presentation. Loid A.

Ongoing Research & Audit

- Title of audit – currently completing the audit loop
  Brief description of audit

- Title of research – currently analysing and interpreting data
  Brief description of audit

Volunteer Work

- Royal National Institute of Blind People: local branch volunteer helper

- Unite For Sight: 3-week volunteer work in India
  Describe your experience and what you learnt

Teaching Experience

- Journal club: Presented in monthly local journal club meetings, (Date)
- Tutorials: Ophthalmic history taking for medical students, (Date)
- Podcast: Glaucoma, University of Edinburgh Medical School, (Date)
- Practice guideline: Assisted in the drafting of the management pathway for orbital cellulitis, Royal Infirmary of Edinburgh (Date)

Management Experience

- 3rd Year Representative, University of Edinburgh Medical School
- University of Edinburgh Medical School representative of the British Undergraduate Ophthalmology Society (BUOS), (Date)

Computing Skills

- Microsoft Office desktop applications software – proficient
- Internet literature search using PubMed and OVID – competent
- SPSS statistical analysis software – competent

Miscellaneous Skills

- Language: Fluent in English and (other languages)
  Interpreted for patients unable to communicate in English

- Driving license: Clean British driving license
- Stereopsis: 60 degrees of arc

Activities & Interests

- Sports: Badminton – played competitively at university level
- Music: Grade 7 piano

Referees

- Mr / Ms / Dr (Name)   (Contact details)
  Local Eye Department

- Professor (Name):   (Contact details)
  Moorfields Eye Hospital:

- Professor (Name):   (Contact details)
  Wills Eye Hospital

Example Questions for OST1 Applications

- Why are you motivated to pursue a career in this specialty? In what way are you able to demonstrate that your own skills and attributes are suitable for a career in this specialty?

- What plan have you followed to develop your understanding of this specialty? How have your actions developed your insight into this specialty?

- Provide evidence of activities / achievements over and above your regular daily activities that demonstrate your personal commitment to this specialty. Indicate date and place relating to the evidence.

- Describe a situation when applying your clinical judgement had a significant impact on patient health. What did you do and how did your judgement contribute to patient health?

- Describe your understanding of medical research to a trainee doctor. You may use examples to illustrate your answer, either from your own experience or from publications if you have not had the opportunity to be involved in research.

- Additional qualifications, prizes, awards, distinctions

- Publications, presentations / posters at conferences

- What experience of delivering teaching do you have?

- What experience of clinical audit do you have? Please state when and where and clearly indicate your level of involvement.

- Describe a time when you had to explain a complex term or procedure to someone. What were the main challenges and the strategies you used?

- Describe a time when a patient had a strong reaction to a diagnosis. Why do you think this was and how did you manage it?

- Describe a recent example of when you have worked as part of a team with other professionals to achieve a specific objective. What approach did you take and how did your actions influence the outcome?

- Provide a specific example of a work situation where professional integrity was required on your part. What approach did you take and how did your actions demonstrate integrity?

Example Standard Interview Questions

General background, CV, application form

- Tell us about yourself
- What is exceptional about your CV?

  (*Note: It will be very embarrassing not to know your CV well, and NEVER lie because it is just not worth it*)

Personal qualities, motivation, drive

- What is your career ambition?
- How do you see yourself in 5 to 10 years' time?

  (*Note: For the academic interview, this is the perfect opportunity to show off your understanding of the academic pathway*)
- Why ophthalmology?
- Convince us of your capability and talent as an ophthalmologist
- How do you know you are making the right career choice?
- What do you have to offer us?
- What are your strengths and weaknesses?

  (*Note: Always dress up your weakness as a form of strength*)

Communication, teamwork, leadership, stress, conflict resolution

- Give us an example where your communication skills made a difference to patient care
- Give us an example where you failed to communicate appropriately
- Give us an example where poor communication resulted in an adverse outcome or near miss
- What are the attributes of a good team player?
- Describe a situation where you showed leadership
- What is the difference between a manager and a leader?
- Tell us a situation where you had conflicts with your colleagues
- How do you handle a non-performing colleague?
- How do you cope with stress?
- How do you cope with having a complaint made against you?

Research and audit

- Tell us about your most recent research
- Tell us about a recent piece of research that has made an impression on you, and why
- Do you think research should be compulsory for all trainees?
- Why is research important?
- What is the difference between audit and research?
- Tell us about the audit cycle
- Why is audit important?
- How can we ensure that audit remains clinically relevant?
- What are the different levels of evidence available?
- What is evidence-based medicine?

Teaching, training, learning, keeping up to date, seeking help

- Tell us about your teaching experience
- What teaching methods do you know?
- What are the pros and cons of problem-based learning?
- What measures do you take to improve your training?
- What is the biggest mistake you have made in a clinical setting?
- How do you keep your skills up-to-date during your research break?

Ethical issues, difficult work scenarios

- Have you ever experienced a difficult work scenario, and how did you deal with it?
- What would you do if you suspected that your consultant has an alcohol or drink-related problem?
- How do you react to your consultant who has mentioned something wrong to a patient?
- What would you do if your consultant goes against protocol?
  (*Note: Always go back to the basic principles: beneficence, justice, respect for autonomy, and non-maleficence*)

Clinical governance and other NHS issues

- What do you know about clinical governance?
- What is evidence-based medicine?
- How do you incorporate evidence-based medicine into your practice?
- What is continuous professional development?
- Why is continuous professional development important?
- What is the difference between assessment and appraisal?
- Tell me about revalidation
- What is the difference between a protocol and a guideline?
- Tell me about the European Working Time Directive (EWTD)
- What is a near miss situation?
- Describe a near miss situation that you have experienced, and how you dealt with the situation
- What is clinical risk management?
- Tell me how you incorporate risk management into your practice
- Tell me about the National Institute of Clinical Excellence (NICE) guidelines regarding (topic)
- Describe the General Medical Council (GMC) good medical practice

Academic interview

- Tell me about your academic experience
- Why become an academic rather than an NHS consultant?
- What are the challenges faced by academic consultants?
- How do you apply for research funding?
- What are the types of professorships?
- Summarise your research in one sentence for the BBC
- Why did you apply for this particular Academic Clinical Fellowship?
- What is the importance of academic medicine?
  (Read the Walport Report to have an understanding of this topic: http://www.nihrtcc.nhs.uk/intetacatrain/index_html/copy_of_Medically_and_Dentally-qualified_Academic_Staff_Report.pdf)

Example Stations for OST1 Interviews

Below are some examples of previous OST1 interview questions when interviews were still conducted by the individual Postgraduate Deaneries.

Deanery 1 (OST1)

- Station 1   -   30 minutes to critically appraise a scientific paper, and then to prepare a 5-minute presentation on it

- Station 2   -   Suturing
  - Fundoscopy and discussion of the clinical findings (e.g. proliferative diabetic retinopathy)

- Station 3   -   Experience of formal and informal teaching
  - Audit cycle and discussion of previously performed audit, including audit outcome
  - Discussion of research experience

- Station 4   -   Critical appraisal of a scientific paper
  - Discussion of publication and general statistics

- Station 5   -   Discussion of portfolio and CV
  - Scenario: *"If your colleague did not turn up at the end of your 12-hour shift, what would you do"*

Deanery 2 (OST1)

- Station 1   -   15 minutes to critically appraise a scientific paper
  - Discussion of the appraisal of the scientific paper
  - Scenario: *"You turned up to clinic with 25 patients and was informed that your Consultant was unable to come to clinic. What would you do?"*

- Station 2   -   Suturing
  - Role play: *"The mother of your 12-year old patient has attended clinic and you suspect a non-organic cause of her visual loss."*
  - Discussion of portfolio and CV

Deanery 3 (OST1)

- Station 1
  - Discussion of portfolio and CV
  - Discussion of a clinical condition (e.g. cataract)
  - Clinical scenario: *"What would you say to a patient who has just been diagnosed with choroidal melanoma?"*
  - Scenario: *"The patient that was booked in for your laser list has informed you that he does not want a junior performing his laser. What would you do?"*

- Station 2
  - Ethical issues related to ophthalmology
  - Discussion of clinical governance

Deanery 4 (OST1)

- Station 1
  - 60 minutes to answer clinical knowledge questions and critically appraise a paper

- Station 2
  - Discussion of the clinical knowledge questions

- Station 3
  - Critical appraisal of the scientific paper
  - Discussion of research experience

- Station 4
  - Scenario: *"What was your worst surgical experience and how did you deal with it?"*

Deanery 5 (OST1)

- Station 1
  - Discussion of portfolio and CV
  - Discussion of personal development

- Station 2
  - Suturing

- Station 3
  - Discussion of common clinical conditions
  - Discussion of research and audit experience

Deanery 6 (OST1)

- Station 1 - 20 minutes to critically appraise a scientific paper, and to prepare presentation on it

- Station 2 - Clinical scenario: *"How would you manage optic neuritis and what would you say to the patient?"*
  - Clinical scenario: *"How would you manage corneal ulcers?"*

- Station 3 - Discussion of good medical practice
  - Discussion of career plans

- Station 4 - Critical appraisal of the scientific paper
  - Discussion of paper and general statistics

Deanery 7 (OST1)

- Station 1 - Interpretation of ophthalmic clinical case notes

- Station 2 - Interpretation of MRI scans

- Station 3 - Suturing

- Station 4 - Role play: *"Breaking bad news: your patient has an ocular tumour and needs an enucleation".*

- Station 5 - Role play: *"You are on-call, and you have to telephone a consultant in the middle of the night to discuss a case."*

- Station 6 - Discussion of Advanced Life Support (ALS)

- Station 7 - Written assessment: Critical thinking, prioritisation of action and utilisation of resources in a difficult clinical scenario

- Station 8 - Discussion of portfolio and CV
  - Discussion of common clinical conditions
  - Discussion of evidence-based medicine

Example Stations for OST2 Interviews

Below are some examples of previous OST2 interview questions when interviews were still conducted by the individual Postgraduate Deaneries.

Deanery 1 (OST2)

- Station 1   -   25 minutes to critically appraise a scientific paper

- Station 2   -   Scenario: *"How would you obtain consent from a patient for a procedure?"*
  - Role play: *"Your patient has been diagnosed with eyelid basal cell carcinoma and would like the diagnosis and management options explained."*

- Station 3   -   Discussion of the critical appraisal of the scientific paper
  - Discussion of research and audit

- Station 4   -   Performing phacoemulsification cataract surgery in a pig eye

- Station 5   -   Discussion of career plans
  - *"Why are you suitable for this job?"*
  - *"What have you done in the last year to support this?"*
  - Scenario: *"How and when would you implement change in the NHS? For instance, using disposable tonometer heads to improve infection control."*
  - *"Do you think you should be more involved in research?"*

Deanery 2 (OST2)

- Station 1 - Clinical scenario: *"Your patient has just been diagnosed with glaucoma, and would like to discuss this with you."*

- Station 2 - Scenario: *"How you deal with difficult colleagues"*

- Station 3 - Scenario: *"Would you see a patient at 3 a.m. in the morning if (different scenarios given)?"*

- Station 4 - Discussion of career plans
  - *"What do you challenging in cataract surgery?"*

- Station 5 - Role play: *"Explaining cataract surgery to a patient."*

Deanery 3 (OST2)

- Station 1 - Scenario: *"How do you consent for cataract surgery?"*
  - Scenario: *"What would you do if you had a dropped nucleus during cataract surgery?"*
  - Scenario: *"The dropped nucleus occurred because the needle was attached correctly to the Healon syringe. Who is to blame?"*
  - Scenario: *"Would you apologise to the patient because of the dropped nucleus?"*
  - Scenario: *"Would you fill in a clinical incident form for dropping the nucleus?"*

- Station 2 - *"Why do you want to do ophthalmology?"*
  - Discussion of teaching experience
  - Discussion of research and audit experience
  - Clinical photograph and discussion of the management options and prognosis (e.g. toxoplasma chorioretinitis)

Glossary

- **Adverse Event**

  Any unfavourable medical occurrence in a patient that resulted in harm
  There are 5 grades of adverse events:
  - *Grade 1: Mild adverse event*
  - *Grade 2: Moderate adverse event*
  - *Grade 3: Severe adverse event*
  - *Grade 4: Life-threatening or disabling adverse event*
  - *Grade 5: Death related to adverse event*

- **Appraisal**

  Process through which opportunities for personal and professional development can be identified and addressed, including discussion of strengths and weaknesses.

- **Assessment**

  Process of evaluating clinical skills or knowledge to see if competency has been achieved in a particular subject and to see if training has been appropriate.

- **Audit**

  "To find out if what you are doing meets the gold standard for high quality healthcare"
  Process where clinical practice or delivery of healthcare is measured against a gold standard, evaluated for deficiencies, and assessed for opportunities for improvement. The audit cycle comprises 5 steps:
  - *Preparation, including selection of care area to be audited*
  - *Criteria selection, including definition of the gold standard*
  - *Data collection and analysis*
  - *Implementation of changes to correct any deficiencies*
  - *Repeating the audit cycle to ensure standard has been met*

- **Clinical Effectiveness**

  "Doing the right thing for the right patient at the right time in the right place"

  Ensuring that high quality clinical care is delivered to provide the best outcomes for the patient.

- **Clinical Governance**

  A framework through which NHS organisations are accountable for continually improving the quality of their services and safeguarding high standards of care by creating an environment in which excellence in clinical care will flourish. The 7 pillars of clinical governance are:
  - *Audit*
  - *Clinical effectiveness and research*
  - *Education and training*
  - *Information and information technology*
  - *Patient and public involvement*
  - *Risk management*
  - *Staffing and staff management*

- **Clinical Practice Guideline**

  Systematically developed statements to assist health care professionals in making clinical decisions to optimise patient care based on specific circumstances, and usually include an assessment of the benefits and harms of alternative care options.

- **Continuous Professional Development**

  Structured and lifelong approach to learning to ensure competence to practice and to keep up to date with skills and knowledge.

- **Critical appraisal**

  Method of assessing and interpreting evidence by carefully and systematically considering its methodology, validity, results and relevance to the area of work being studied.

- **European Working Time Directive (EWTD)**
  http://ec.europa.eu/social/main.jsp?catId=706&langId=en&intPageId=205
  Ruling to protect workers' health and safety, and specifies that each European Union member state must ensure workers are entitled to:
  - *Weekly working time less than 48 hours on average, including overtime*
  - *Minimum daily rest period of 11 consecutive hours every 24 hours*
  - *Rest break during working time if duty is longer than 6 hours*
  - *Minimum weekly rest period of 24 uninterrupted hours every 7 days*
  - *Paid annual leave of at least 4 weeks per year*
  - *Extra protection for night work*

- **Evidence-Based Medicine**
  "Using best evidence to make clinical decisions for the patient"
  Process of systematically reviewing, appraising and using clinical research to aid delivery of optimum clinical care to patients. The evidence is graded in 4 levels (there are other grading schemes):
  - *Level A: Randomised clinical trial; Systematic meta-analysis*
  - *Level B: Case-control study*
  - *Level C: Case series*
  - *Level D: Case report; Expert opinion*

- **Good Medical Practice**
  http://www.gmc-uk.org/guidance/good_medical_practice/contents.asp
  Describes the behaviour and judgement to practise in a way that would meet standards expected by peers, the community, and the General Medical Council. It comprises 4 domains:
  - *Domain 1: Knowledge, skills and performance*
  - *Domain 2: Safety and quality*
  - *Domain 3: Communication, partnership and teamwork*
  - *Domain 4: Maintaining trust*

- **National Institute of Clinical Excellence (NICE)**

  http://www.nice.org.uk

  Organisation responsible for providing national guidance (through NICE guidelines) on the promotion of good health and the prevention and treatment of ill health, to ensure care provided is of the best possible quality and best value for money.

- **National Patient Safety Agency (NPSA)**

  http://www.npsa.nhs.uk

  Organisation responsible for improving patient safety by monitoring and recording patient safety incidents, and by supporting and influencing organisations working in the healthcare sector.

- **National Service Frameworks (NSFs)**

  http://www.nhs.uk/nhsengland/NSF/pages/Nationalserviceframeworks.aspx

  Policies set by the NHS to define clear quality requirements of care for major medical conditions such as cancer, coronary heart disease and diabetes, based on best available evidence of what treatments and services work most effectively for patients.

- **Near miss**

  An unplanned event that did not cause harm to the patient, but had the potential to do so.

- **Patient Advice and Liaison Service (PALS)**

  Service providing confidential advice, information and support for patients, carers and families.

- **Protocol**

  Pre-defined written plan, developed from evidence based medicine, which forms the standard of care in the management of a particular medical condition or situation.

- **Research**

  "To find out if there are better ways of delivering healthcare and achieving better outcomes"

  The systematic and scientific investigation into aspects of medicine and healthcare (including basic science, epidemiology and clinical trials) in order to establish facts and reach new conclusions.

- **Revalidation**

  http://www.gmc-uk.org/doctors/revalidation.asp

  Process for doctors licensed to practise in the UK to prove that their skills and knowledge are up to date and that they remain fit to practise medicine in their chosen specialty. This occurs every 5 years, and encompasses following 6 areas:
  - *Continuing professional development*
  - *Quality improvement activity*
  - *Significant events*
  - *Feedback from colleagues*
  - *Feedback from patients*
  - *Review of complaints and compliments*

- **Risk Management**

  "To minimise risk of adverse events and near misses to the patient"

  The process of having robust systems to understand, monitor, record, and minimise risk to patients and healthcare professionals during healthcare delivery. This includes:
  - *Identification of adverse events and near misses during care*
  - *Understanding factors that influence the occurrence of adverse events*
  - *Reporting of adverse events, e.g. through critical incident forms*
  - *Learning lessons from adverse events*
  - *Prevention of adverse events from recurring Implementation of steps to reduce the risk of adverse events*
  - *Promotion of a blame-free culture*

Conclusion

A career in ophthalmology is very fulfilling, satisfying and definitely worthwhile pursuing. You will not regret it. It provides the best combination of cutting edge surgery, medical advancement, imaging technology, and excellent quality of life. However, there are no short cuts. The initial road can be long and difficult, but do persevere and work hard. Try and try again... and along the way obtain feedback on how you can improve. The initial stumbling block may prove insurmountable. But don't think of past failures as such; they are but learning experiences to set you on your way to success. Something becomes a problem only when your mind perceives it as such. So always **THINK POSITIVE!** After you edge past the first hurdle, you notice that things get easier. Opportunities come by more easily. More and more colleagues approach you for collaborations in research projects, audits and presentations. You meet more mentors in various settings. Your CV grows impressively. Interview shortlistings become more frequent. And eventually you WILL secure that coveted ophthalmology training post!

So what are you waiting for?

To Your Success in Ophthalmology!

Brian Ang
Shi Zhuan Tan
Ken Lee Lai
http://ophthalmologytraining.blogspot.com

About the Authors

Brian (Ghee Soon) Ang MBChB, FRCOphth, FRANZCO is a Consultant Ophthalmologist at the Glaucoma Unit of the Royal Victorian Eye & Ear Hospital in Melbourne, Australia. He completed his ophthalmology training in the United Kingdom as a Specialist Registrar in Aberdeen, and furthered his glaucoma training in Geneva, Switzerland and Wellington, New Zealand. He is actively involved in the teaching and training of medical students, optometrists, allied health professionals and junior ophthalmologists. He has published over 50 peer-reviewed scientific articles and is a reviewer for the UK National Institute for Health Research, and for ophthalmology journals such as Ophthalmology, British Journal of Ophthalmology, Eye, Clinical & Experimental Ophthalmology, and Journal of Glaucoma. He currently serves as a member of the Associate Advisory Committee for the International Society of Glaucoma Surgery and the Expert Advisory Panel for Glaucoma Australia, and is the webmaster for www.vision-and-eye-health.com.

Shi Zhuan Tan MBChB is an Academic Specialty Trainee in Ophthalmology in Manchester (North Western Deanery). She graduated from the University of Edinburgh in 2008, and has a strong interest in research and academic ophthalmology.

Ken Lee Lai MBChB graduated from the University of Edinburgh, and is currently an Ophthalmology Specialty Trainee in Glasgow (West of Scotland Deanery). He is a keen advocate for charity work, and has already contributed to a Unite for Sight charity programme in India.

Made in the USA
Charleston, SC
08 February 2014